Heino Kienapfel

Klaus-Dieter Kühn

(Eds.)

The Infected Implant

Heino Kienapfel
Klaus-Dieter Kühn

(Eds.)

The Infected Implant

With 98 Figures and 16 Tables

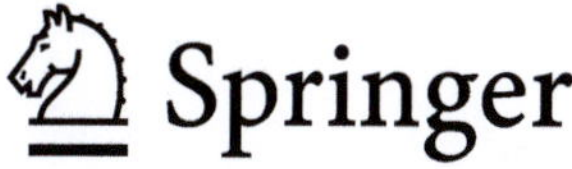

Prof. Dr. med. Heino Kienapfel
Vivantes Auguste - Viktoria - Klinik
Dept. of Special Orthopeadic Surgery and
Traumatology
Centre of Joint Arthroplasty
Rubensstr. 125
12157 Berlin
Germany

Dr. rer. nat. Klaus-Dieter Kühn
Heraeus Medical GmbH
Philipp-Reis Str. 8/13
61273 Wehrheim
Germany

This book and the basic Symposium in Potsdam, November 21–22, 2008 have been sponsored by
Heraeus Medical GmbH, Wehrheim.
Cover image: Scanning electron micrograph of *Staphylococcus aureus* biofilm adhered to a metal implant surface.
Taken by Dr Llinos G Harris, Medical Microbiology, Institute of Life Science, School of Medicine, Swansea University,
Swansea, SA2 8PP, Wales, UK.

ISBN 978-3-540-92835-5 Springer Medizin Verlag Heidelberg

Bibliografische Information der Deutschen Bibliothek
The Deutsche Bibliothek lists this publication in Deutsche Nationalbibliographie;
detailed bibliographic data is available in the internet at http://dnb.ddb.de.

Springer Medizin Verlag
springer.com
© Springer Medizin Verlag Heidelberg 2009

Planning: Hanna Hensler-Fritton, Heidelberg
Projectmanagement: Diana Kraplow, Heidelberg
Copy-Editing: Hilger Verlagsservice, Heidelberg
Design: deblik Berlin
Typesetting: TypoStudio Tobias Schaedla, Heidelberg
Printer: Stürtz GmbH, Würzburg

SPIN: 12586806

Printed on acid free paper   18/5135/DK – 5 4 3 2 1 0

Foreword

Infections following joint arthroplasty are a severe complication for each patient with a negative impact on their quality of life. Infections are also a challenge for the surgeons, microbiologists and hospitals involved. Finally, due to their financial impact infections will increasingly be monitored and controlled, as they have a direct influence on how hospitals will be reimbursed; as such, preventing infections has been identified as a source of cost reduction. Furthermore, the issue of infection needs to be a standard part of any outcome measurement – be it based on information obtained from registers or from patient reported outcome studies / questionnaires. The goal of the 2nd International Arthroplasty Symposium – The Infected Implant of November 21–22, 2008 in Potsdam was to provide an expert update on the state of the art, with regard to the basic knowledge on and clinical treatment options for this patient group.

We would like to thank all the presenters for their contributions to this book. Among the topics you will find valuable information on: basic science, epidemiology, microbiology, documentation in orthopaedic surgery and on, surgical as well as local and systemic drug therapy algorithms.

We hope that this book will help us all to further improve the treatment quality and outcome for our patients.

Klaus-Dieter Kühn
Heino Kienapfel

Table of Contents

List of Contributors

Aliprandi, Alberto
Radiology Department, Università degli Studi
di Milano, Via Festa del Perdono 7, 20122 Milano,
ITALY

Babiak, Ireneusz
Department of Orthopaedics and Traumatology of
the Locomotor System Medical University of Warsaw,
POLAND

Banci, Lorenzo
Hip Department – Centro di Chirurgia dell'Anca,
Via Lusardi 5, 20122 Milano, ITALY

Bauer, Thomas
Department of Orthopedic Surgery, Ambroise Paré
University Hospital, 9 Avenue Charles de Gaulle,
92100 Boulogne, FRANCE

Cordero-Ampuero, José
University Hospital La Princesa, Universidad
Autónoma de Madrid, c/Océano Antártico 41,
Tres Cantos, 28760 Madrid, SPAIN

Eberhardt, Christian
University Hospital Frankfurt, Department Orthope-
dic Surgery, Marienburgstraße 2, 60528 Frankfurt,
GERMANY

Engesæter, Lars B.
Norwegian Arthroplasty Register, University of
Bergen, Department of Orthopedic Surgery,
Möllendalsbakken 11, 5021 Bergen, NORWAY

Foerster, Götz von
Tabea-Krankenhaus, Artemed-Kliniken GmbH,
Kösterbergstraße 32, 22587 Hamburg, GERMANY

Frommelt, Lars
ENDO-Klinik Hamburg – Service for Infectious
Diseases, Clinical Microbiology and Infection Control,
Holstenstraße 2, 22767 Hamburg, GERMANY

Gaiser, Sebastian
Heraeus Medical GmbH, Philipp-Reis-Straße
8/13, 61273 Wehrheim, GERMANY

Górecki, Andrzeij
Department of Orthopaedics and Traumatology of
the Locomotor System Medical University of Warsaw,
POLAND

Jahoda, David
Department of Orthopaedics, 1st Faculty of Medicine,
Teaching Hospital Motol, V Úvalu 84, 15006 Prague 5,
CZECH REPUBLIC

Kärrholm, Johan
Department of Orthopaedics, Sahlgrenska University
Hospital, PO Box 100, 40530 Gothenburg, SWEDEN

Krbec, Martin
Orthopaedic Dpt. of University Hospital, Masaryk
University, Jihlavská 20, 62500 Brno, CZECH REPUBLIC

Lortat-Jacob, Alain
Department of Orthopedic Surgery, Ambroise Paré
University Hospital, 9 Avenue Charles de Gaulle,
92100 Boulogne, FRANCE

Lubinus, Philipp
Special Department Endoprothetics, Lubinus
Clinicum, Steenbeker Weg 25, 24106 Kiel, GERMANY

Luňáček, Libor
Orthopaedic and Traumatological Clinic, Charles University, Celetná 13, 11000 Praha 1, CZECH REPUBLIC

Meani, Enzo
Osteoarticular Infection Surgery Unit, Istituto
Ortopedico Gaetano Pini, Piazza Ferrari Andrea 1,
20122 Milano, ITALY

Randelli, Filippo
Hip Department – Centro di Chirurgia dell'Anca,
Via Lusardi 5, 20122 Milano, ITALY

Robertsson, Otto

Department of Orthopaedics, Lund University
Hospital, 22185 Lund, SWEDEN

Rodloff, Arne C.

Institute for Medical Microbiology and Epidemiology
of Infectious Diseases, University of Leipzig,
Liebigstraße 24, 04103 Leipzig, GERMANY

Sardanelli, Francesco

Radiology Department, Università degli Studi di
Milano, Via Festa del Perdono 7, 20122 Milano, ITALY

Sauer, Joachim

DP-Medsystems AG, Tulpenstr. 26, 82110 Germering,
GERMANY

Schaumann, Reiner

Institute for Medical Microbiology and Epidemiology
of Infectious Diseases, University of Leipzig,
Liebigstraße 24, 04103 Leipzig, GERMANY

Sconfienza, Luca

Radiology Department, Università degli Studi di
Milano, Via Festa del Perdono 7, 20122 Milano, ITALY

Stefánsdóttir, Anna

Department of Orthopaedics, Lund University
Hospital, 22185 Lund, SWEDEN

Stockley, Ian

Department for Orthopaedics, Northern General
Hospital, Herries Road, Sheffield, South Yorkshire,
S5 7AU, UNITED KINGDOM

Trezza, Paolo

Osteoarticular Infection Surgery Unit, Istituto
Ortopedico Gaetano Pini, Piazza Ferrari Andrea 1,
20122 Milano, ITALY

Vansintjan, Pieter

Department of Orthopaedic Surgery, Stedelijk Zieken-
huis, Brugsesteenweg 90, 8800 Roeselare, BELGIUM

Verdonk, Peter C.M.

Department of Orthopaedic Surgery, Ghent University
Hospital, De Pintelaan 185, 9000 Ghent, BELGIUM

Verdonk, René

Department of Orthopaedic Surgery, Ghent University
Hospital, De Pintelaan 185, 9000 Ghent, BELGIUM

Zahár, Ákos

Semmelweis University, Department of Orthopaedics,
Karolina út 27, 1113 Budapest XI, HUNGARY

The Importance of European Registers in Respect to Infections in Arthroplasty

Ákos Zahár

In surgery, especially in orthopaedic surgery, quality control is one of the main tools to gain feedback of the surgeon's activity for healthcare professionals. The results from our daily activity, the outcome of the surgical procedures are widely published in the scientific literature and in on-line versions of our peer-reviewed journals. Statistical analysis of the data from the scientific works and meta-analyses created from them are major tools to have information of our surgical activity, or to get knowledge about the quality of orthopaedic devices we are using.

The legal aspect of documentation is nowadays obvious for every practicing surgeon. The accurate documentation of each and every patient who underwent a procedure is essential in legal affaires. Also national healthcare systems use the data of our scientific or statistical databases, that is why the financial impact of documentation is enormous.

Establishing arthroplasty registers in the late 1970's – the first ever was the Swedish Knee Arthroplasty Register in 1975 – had also the goal to improve quality of orthopaedic surgical activity in order to rule out implants with clinically poor results. The output was that the revision burden of the implants – both hip and knee – decreased significantly. The publication of the results from the Swedish Arthroplasty Register could be widely used in all over the world. Another result of the Swedish model was that other countries, first of all Scandinavian countries followed the Swedish example.

Recent publications of the Swedish Arthroplasty Register report that the cemented technique is the dominating type of fixation throughout Sweden. Infection prophylaxis is achieved in both ways: systemic and local application of antibiotics is widely used. The septic revision rate after total hip arthroplasty (THA) is about 0.6%, which is an enormous improvement compared to the data of the past decade. Furthermore, the colleagues from Sweden report that MRSA is fortunately not yet an issue in Scandinavia.

Norway started its register in 1987, it was a surveillance tool to identify inferior implants as early as possible – as we can read in the Mission Statement of the Norwegian Arthroplasty Register. Colleagues from Norway could detect products like PMMA bone cements with poor survival rates. So the products with high failure rates could be eliminated from the national market. Nowadays the Norwegian group of register professionals has gained the title National Centre of Excellence – 98% of all THA are reported in the Register.

The data from Norway reveal that the number of uncemented THA decreases, while hybrid technique is increasing. The use of bone cement without antibiotics disappeared in the last 5 years. Local and systemic antibiotic prophylaxis is used in Norway, but systemic antibiotic is administered on a four-times-a-day basis for 24 hours. Increasing number of revisions due to infection are reported in the Norwegian Register, the true causes are being explained.

The financial impact of the Scandinavian registers was that the expenses for the establishment of a national register were compared to those of avoidable revision surgeries. Based upon these findings, further financial support could be achieved by the healthcare systems, as experienced recently in Romania.

The Scandinavian experience made it possible to build up further arthroplasty registers in the European countries. One of the first non-Scandinavian countries was Hungary, which joined the family of national registers in 1998. The success in the funding of a nation-wide register is highly dependent from its strong regulations, compact and effective organisation. The comparability of the national results is achieved by a minimum dataset of arthroplasty registers, which was introduced by the European Arthroplasty Register (EAR).

The financial support of each national arthroplasty register varies from country to country. There is a wide range between the amounts depending on the engagement of the national healthcare system, ministry of health and other official federal or governmental institutions. There are countries, where the government supports the work of registers, like Austria, Romania, and there are other countries, where the financial support is an obligation of the national orthopaedic society together with manufacturers of orthopaedic implants.

An effective system on a country level is only achieved if all orthopaedic and trauma centres are involved, sufficient financial support is secured, and the healthcare system is highly dedicated to obtain data from the national register.

The European Federation of Orthopaedic and Trauma Surgery (EFORT) started the EAR project in 2002 with the goal to collect data from the national registers in the EU, in order to improve the quality of orthopaedic implants throughout Europe. Co-operation agreements with all national arthroplasty registers make it possible to achieve the highest level of osteoarthritis treatment. The EAR is about to introduce new regulatory requirements for implants in the EU.

The publication raising from the data collected in arthroplasty registers are available in annual reports (Sweden, Norway, Denmark) or in peer-reviewed journals. They are available for everybody in the internet portals of each national register.

Treatment guidelines also belong to the topic of documentation, even though if they suggest a sequence of diagnostic and therapeutic tools. The algorithm of managing periprosthetic infections is very useful in daily practice, even if the orthopaedic surgeon has to deal with highly demanding cases. Standardisation of treatment options in form of a defined algorithm helps to improve the quality of treatment and to avoid failures. The publications in peer-reviewed journals are only recommendations, while nation-wide regulations like treatment guidelines are mandatory for healthcare professionals.

In a well-defined treatment algorithm we can choose the proper option from the different solutions: debridement without exchange, one-stage exchange, two-stage revision with or without antibiotic spacer etc. Recurrence of the infection can be kept on a very low rate (under 5%) when we follow the instructions of the Swiss colleagues (The Liestal Algorithm).

Documentation and to share information in the cases of infected implants are of great importance. The distribution of causative agents, like *Staphylococcus aureus* and *Coagulase-negative Staphylococci,* are highly interesting data for both infectologists and orthopaedic surgeons. Polyresistant strains like MRSE and MRSA are also reported in arthroplasty registers in order to be prepared for the increasing number of cases. The results of local and systemic antibiotic prophylaxis are well known from the annual reports of Sweden and Norway. Publications of novel treatment options, like new drugs in chemotherapy, local application of antibiotics or improved antimicrobial coatings, belong to the topics of documentation, too.

Increasing Incidence of Infected THA in Norway Despite Improved Antibiotic Prophylaxis

Lars B. Engesæter

Introduction

In orthopaedic implant surgery, infection is rare but devastating for the patient and costly for society. With improved surgical techniques, stricter pre- and perioperative routines and antibiotic prophylaxis, the infection rate after primary total hip arthroplasty (THA) has been reduced from 5–10% in the late 1960s to around 1% today (Lidgren 2001; Lidgren et al. 2003; Zimmerli et al. 2004). In previous papers based on the Norwegian Arthroplasty Register, a lower revision rate of primary THAs was found when antibiotic prophylaxis was given both systemically and in the bone cement compared to systemically only, in bone cement only, or compared to no antibiotic prophylaxis at all (Espehaug et al. 1997; Engesaeter et al. 2006). The importance of systemic antibiotic prophylaxis in primary THA surgery seems to be well accepted; however, the benefits of antibiotic prophylaxis in bone cement remain in question (van de Belt et al. 2001).

Based on the data in the Norwegian Arthroplasty Register (NAR), we report in this paper on the use of antibiotic prophylaxis in primary THA and the incidence of reported revisions for infection after primary THAs in the period 1987–2007.

Methods

The Norwegian Arthroplasty Register is a nationwide registry, established in September 1987. Each THA performed in Norway is reported individually by the surgeon by completing a standard form (Havelin et al. 2000). Information on the form includes the identity of the patient, the date of the operation, indication for surgery, type of prosthesis, type of cement, operation time, type of operating room and, if systemic antibiotic prophylaxis was used, the type, duration and dosage. Revision of the implant is defined as surgical removal or change of the whole or part of the implant. Using the unique identification number assigned to each inhabitant of Norway, the information from the primary THA was linked to any eventual revision in the registry.

Survival analyses were performed using the Kaplan-Meier method and the Cox regression model. Relative revision risks (RR) are presented with adjustment for differences among groups in gender, age, cement brand, type of systemic antibiotic prophylaxis, prosthesis type, type of operating theatre, and duration of the operation. The risk for revision due to deep infection was calculated with time stratified into four 5-year periods. Patients who died or emigrated during the follow-up period were identified from files provided by Statistics Norway. The follow-up time for the prostheses in these patients were censored at the date of death or emigration.

Results

Since the start of the Register in September 1987 to the end of December 2007, 110,985 primary THAs have been reported to the NAR. In 1987, 82.8% of patients with primary THA received systemic antibiotic prophylaxis, and 99.5% in 2007. Antibiotics in the cement were used in 36% of the operations in 1987 and in 100% in 2007. We have previously shown that the lowest revision risk was found when antibiotic prophylaxis was given both systemically and in the cement (Engesaeter et al. 2003). Compared to this combined regime, patients who received antibiotic prophylaxis only systemically had a revision rate 1.4 times higher with all reasons for revision as endpoint (p = 0.001), 1.3 times higher with aseptic loosening (p = 0.02) and 1.8 times higher with infection as endpoint in the analyses (p = 0.01) (Fig. 2.1).

For the combined antibiotic regime (antibiotic both systemically and in cement), the results were better if antibiotics were administered four times on the day of surgery compared to once (p < 0.001), twice (p < 0.001) or three times (p = 0.02) (Fig. 2.2). In 2007, systemic antibiotic prophylaxis was given four times on the day of surgery in 77% of the primary THAs compared to 30% for the whole period.

For the whole period 1987–2007, 110,882 primary THAs were reported of which 706 were revised due to infection. This number of primary revisions due to infection is increasing. Compared to the primary THAs implanted in 1987–1992, the risk for revision due to infection was 1.3 times higher for those implanted in 1993–1997 (p = 0.05), 1.4 times higher for 1998–2002 (p = 0.01), and 2.7 times higher for 2003–2007 (p = <0.001). This increase in revisions due to infection was also found when analysing separately for cemented THAs and was even more pronounced for uncemented THAs.

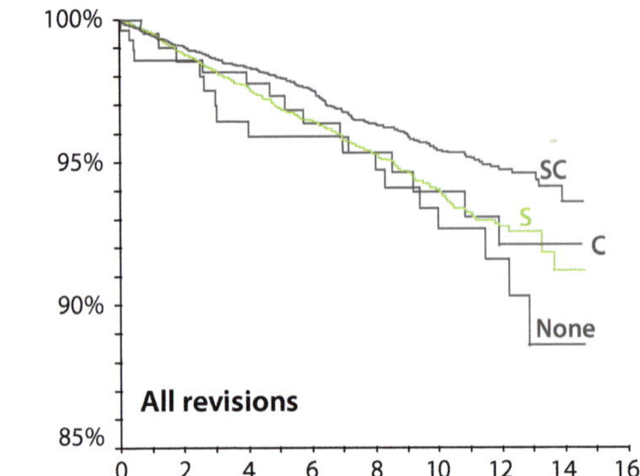

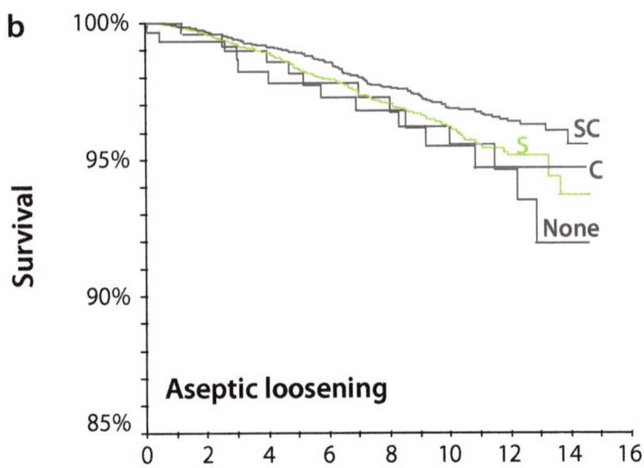

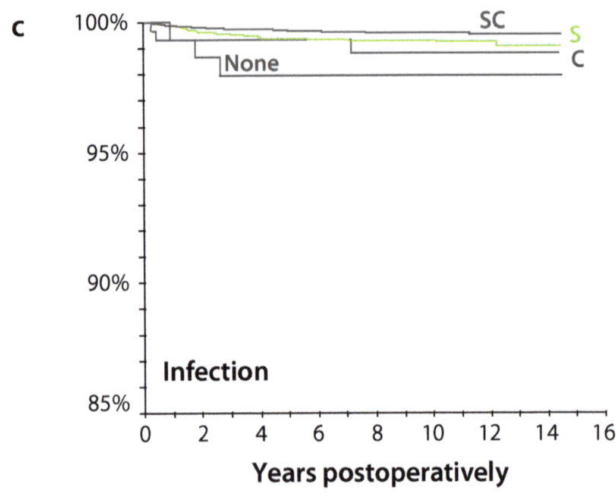

Fig. 2.1a–c. Cox-adjusted survival curves with all reasons for revision (**a**), aseptic loosening (**b**) and infection (**c**) as endpoints for THAs with antibiotic prophylaxis systemically and in cement (*SC*), systemically only (*S*), in cement only (*C*), or no antibiotic prophylaxis (None)

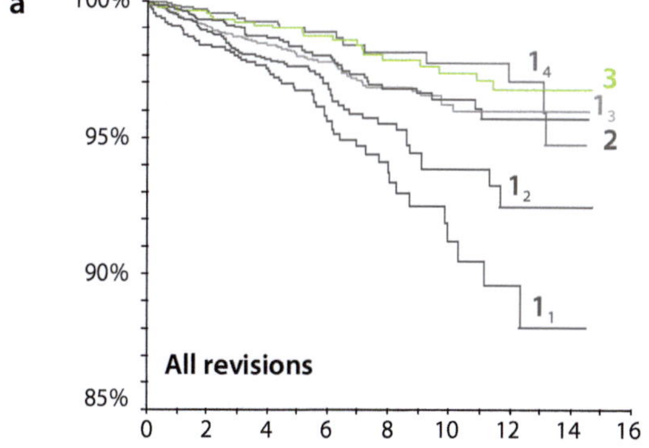

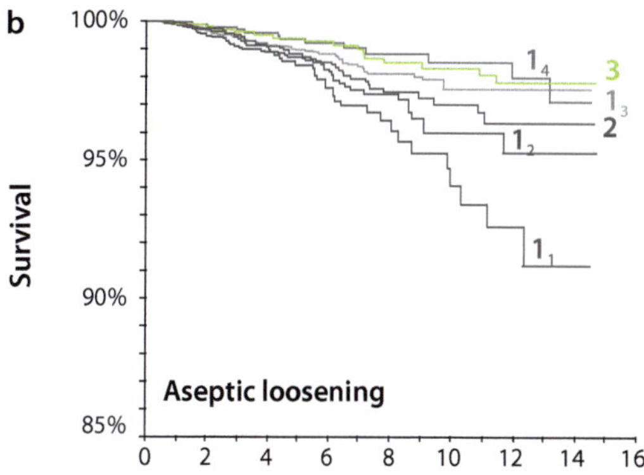

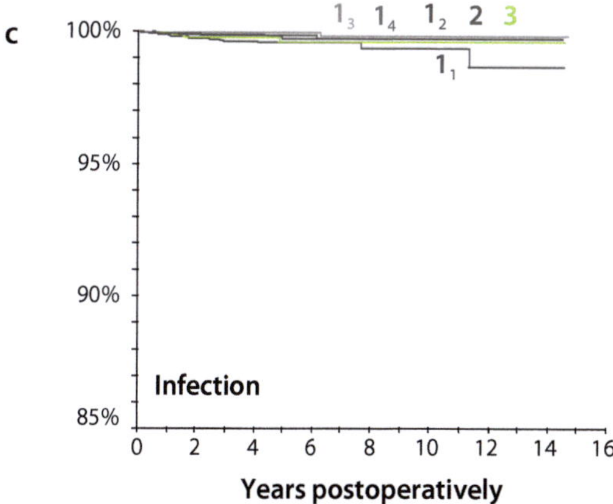

Fig. 2.2a–c. Cox-adjusted survival curves with all reasons for revision (**a**), aseptic loosening (**b**) and infection (**c**) as endpoints for THAs with antibiotic prophylaxis systemically for 1 day (with the number of doses as subscript, i.e. 1 dose (1_1), 2 doses (1_2), 3 doses (1_3) and 4 doses (1_4)), 2 days (2) and 3 days (3) combined with antibiotic in the cement

Discussion

The best results of primary THAs were obtained among those patients who received prophylactic antibiotic both in cement and systemically, and where the systemic antibiotic was given four times on the day of surgery. In the Norwegian Arthroplasty Register the number of reported revisions due to infection after primary THA is, nevertheless, increasing.

However, the explanation for the increase in reported infected THAs to the registry is not straightforward. The possibility that the increase is real can of course not be excluded, a finding also reported by Kurtz et al. (2008). Simultaneous changes in possible confounding factors have occurred, however. For example, in recent years low-grade infections of prostheses have been in focus, both for the orthopaedic surgeon and the microbiologist, with better diagnostics for these infections (Zimmerli and Ochsner 2003). In accordance with this, there has been a decrease in the number of reported aseptic loosenings: it is possible that some infections reported today were earlier reported as aseptic loosenings.

Furthermore, more aggressive surgical treatment of early infected THAs without removal of the implant is now more common. Such revisions without removing or exchanging part of the implants are not reported to the register. With modular prostheses, which have become more common in recent years, easily removable parts are exchanged and accordingly reported to the register. This could also contribute to the increase in reported infections.

It is, however, reassuring for us that our recommendations of four doses of systemic antibiotic prophylaxis on the day of surgery combined with antibiotic in the cement still gives the best survival for primary THAs, with all reasons for revision, with aseptic loosening, and with infection as endpoint in the analyses.

Conclusions

In the Norwegian Arthroplasty Register the best results for primary THA are found when antibiotic prophylaxis is given both systemically and in the bone cement, and if the systemic antibiotic is administered four times on the day of surgery. The number of reported revisions to our registry due to deep infection has, however, increased in recent years without the reasons being evident.

References

Engesaeter LB, Lie SA, Espehaug B, Furnes O, Vollset SE, Havelin LI (2003) Antibiotic prophylaxis in total hip arthroplasty: effects of antibiotic prophylaxis systemically and in bone cement on the revision rate of 22,170 primary hip replacements followed 0–14 years in the Norwegian Arthroplasty Register. Acta Orthop Scand 74: 644–651

Engesaeter LB, Espehaug B, Lie SA, Furnes O, Havelin LI (2006) Does cement increase the risk of infection in primary total hip arthroplasty? Revision rates in 56,275 cemented and uncemented primary THAs followed for 0–16 years in the Norwegian Arthroplasty Register. Acta Orthop 77: 351–358

Espehaug B, Engesaeter LB, Vollset SE, Havelin LI, Langeland N (1997) Antibiotic prophylaxis in total hip arthroplasty. Review of 10,905 primary cemented total hip replacements reported to the Norwegian arthroplasty register, 1987 to 1995. J Bone Joint Surg Br 79: 590–595

Havelin LI, Engesaeter LB, Espehaug B, Furnes O, Lie SA, Vollset SE (2000) The Norwegian Arthroplasty Register: 11 years and 73,000 arthroplasties. Acta Orthop Scand 71: 337–353

Kurtz SM, Lau E, Schmier J, Ong KL, Zhao K, Parvizi J (2008) Infection Burden for Hip and Knee Arthroplasty in the United States. J Arthroplasty 23: 984–991

Lidgren L (2001) Joint prosthetic infections: a success story. Acta Orthop Scand 72: 553–556

Lidgren L, Knutson K, Stefansdottir A (2003) Infection and arthritis. Infection of prosthetic joints. Best Pract Res Clin Rheumatol 17: 209–218

van de Belt H, Neut D, Schenk W, van Horn JR, van der Mei HC, Busscher HJ (2001) Infection of orthopedic implants and the use of antibiotic-loaded bone cements. A review. Acta Orthop Scand 72: 557–571

Zimmerli W, Ochsner PE (2003) Management of infection associated with prosthetic joints. Infection 31: 99–108

Zimmerli W, Trampuz A, Ochsner PE (2004) Prosthetic-joint infections. N Engl J Med 351: 1645–1654

Update from the Swedish Arthroplasty Registers with Special Reference to Infections

Anna Stefánsdóttir, Johan Kärrholm, Otto Robertsson

Introduction

The Swedish Arthroplasty Registers were the first national arthroplasty registers and were initiated by the Swedish Orthopaedic Society. The knee arthroplasty register was established in 1975 and the hip arthroplasty register in 1979. These were the times of rapid development and limited guidance from the literature. The pioneers that started the registers realised that it would be impossible for the individual surgeon to base the choice of optimal operative treatment on his/her own experience. The aim was to give early warning of inferior designs and present average results based on the experience of a whole nation instead of that of highly specialized units (Robertsson et al. 2000). The work performed by the registers has been successful and contributed to continuous improvements in arthroplastic surgery and has inspired orthopaedic surgeons in other countries to start their own national registers. The scope of the Swedish registers have through the years widened and apart from the annual reports, that are available in English version at the websites, www.knee.se and www.jru.orthop.gu.se, research in specific fields have been presented in scientific papers and theses that are listed at the websites. Rare but devastating complications, like deep infection after arthroplastic surgery, can preferably be studied by using data from the national registers.

Material

At present knee arthroplasties are performed at 76 orthopaedic departments and hip arthroplasties at 79 departments, all of them reporting to the national registers (Kärrholm et al. 2007; Robertsson and Lidgren 2008). With the exception of few private hospitals, where reporting to the registers is a prerequisite for payment, the reporting is voluntary. The data is continuously validated and in 2007 96% of primary hip arthroplasties were reported (Kärrholm et al. 2007) and it has been estimated that 94% of knee revisions are accounted for (Robertsson et al. 1999).

The knee arthroplasty register, that is located in Lund and directed by professor Lars Lidgren, contained information on 138,255 primary knee arthroplasties at the end of 2007. Information is collected on special forms that are filled in during surgery and mailed to Lund. Implant stickers are pasted on the forms, which give detailed information and make it possible to track implants. The hip arthroplasty register, that is located in Gothenburg and directed by professor Johan Kärrholm, contained information on 284,630 primary hip arthroplasties at the end of 2007. Information is collected on web-based forms filled in by personal at the operating departments and includes detailed information about the implants. In the case of revision, the information is completed with copies of patient files that are analysed by register personal. During the last decade there has been a shift in Sweden in the treatment of dislocated hip fractures, from closed reduction and internal fixation to hemi-arthroplasty or total hip arthroplasty. Hemi-arthroplasties of the hip have since 2005 been registered in the hip arthroplasty register. This part of the register is directed by Dr. Cecilia Rogmark in Malmö and contained information on 12,245 hemi-arthroplasties at the end of 2007.

The primary outcome variable is revision arthroplasty and the results are presented as implant survival at 5 and 10 years. Revision is defined as any operation including addition, exchange or removal of prosthetic components (including amputation and arthrodesis). Among other outcome variables there is 90-day mortality, gain in quality of life at 1 year follow-up (EQ-5D) and reoperation within 2 years after hip arthroplasty. When comparing groups of patients operated on at different times, account can be taken for differences, for example in age and time of operation, by calculating the cumulative revision rate (CRR).

The yearly number of primary knee and hip arthroplasties has increased enormously (Fig. 3.1

and 3.2) and in 2007 approximately 10,000 primary knee arthroplasties, 14,000 primary hip arthroplasties and 3000 hemi-arthroplasties of the hip

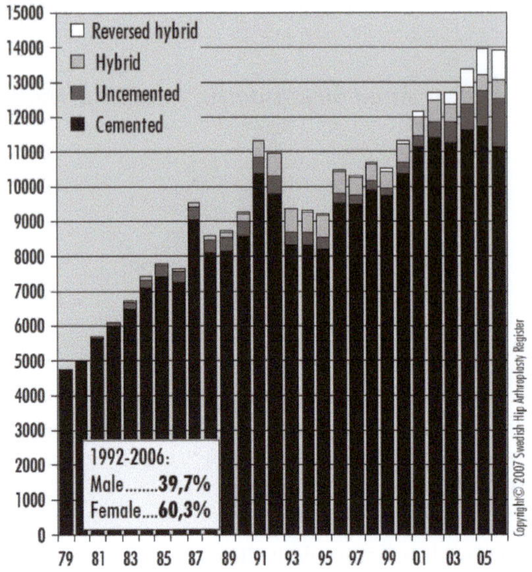

Fig. 3.2. The yearly number of primary hip arthroplasties during 1979 to 2006 divided according to the type of fixation. (Published with permission from the Swedish hip arthroplasty register)

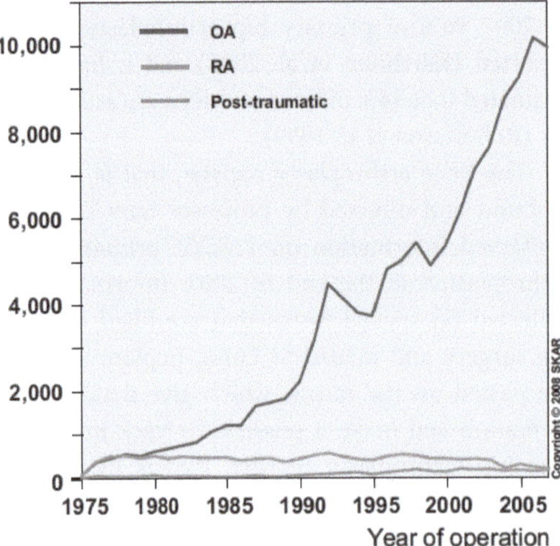

Fig. 3.1. The yearly number of primary knee arthroplasties during 1975 to 2007 divided according to primary diagnosis. (Published with permission from the Swedish knee arthroplasty register)

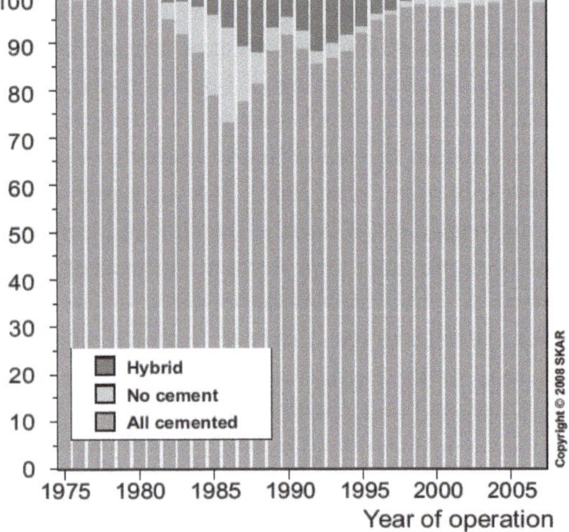

Fig. 3.3. The relative yearly distribution regarding the use of cement for fixation in primary knee arthroplasty during 1975 to 2007. (Published with permission from the Swedish knee arthroplasty register)

were performed. The increase in the number of knee arthroplasties have been faster and is due to the increasing number of patients with osteoarthritis (OA) while the number of patients with rheumatoid arthritis having a knee arthroplasty have decreased.

The dominating type of fixation is with bone-cement (■ Fig. 3.2 and 3.3). In hip arthroplasty the use of uncemented implants has been increasing and in 2007 approximately 20% of the stems and 15% of the cups were uncemented. In Sweden, principally all cement used in hip and knee arthroplasty contains gentamicin.

The systemic antibiotic prophylaxis is not registered in the individual case but recently information was collected about 300 total knee arthroplasties performed during 2007 (unpublished material from the Swedish knee arthroplasty register). 88.7% of the patients received the beta-lactam drug cloxacillin, 9.7% received clindamycin and 1.6% cefuroxim. In the Hip Arthroplasty Register use of antibiotic prophylaxis is recorded per operating department.

Results

Information about the true infection rate after primary hip- and knee arthroplasty is not available as the primary outcome variable in the registers is a revision or reoperation. Those infected patients that for some reason or another are treated only with suppressive antibiotic therapy will not be reported and no information is gathered about infected knee arthroplasties treated with soft-tissue surgery without the change of a prosthetic component. During the years 2003 to 2007 the number of first-time revisions of primary hip- or knee arthroplasty due to infection was fairly constant with the exception of a higher number of infected hip arthroplasties revised in 2007 (■ Table 3.1). During this 5-year period, 740 first-time revisions were performed due to infection, 7777 first-time revisions were performed due to causes other than infection and 116,444 primary hip- and knee arthroplasties were performed.

Infection becomes a more frequent cause of revision for every revision of a hip arthroplasty, in-

fections accounting for 7.4% of first time revisions, 11.9% of second revisions, 14.4% of third time revisions and 21.9% of fourth or more revisions.

Approximately 3% of the patients having a hemi-arthroplasty because of hip fracture had some reoperation during the short follow-up time until the end of 2007. The most common cause of reoperation was dislocation (49.7%), but in second place infection (28.8%) and commonly the infected patients had several reoperations. In this elderly and frail patient population the 90-day mortality was 12%.

The cumulative revision rate because of infection has decreased during the three decades the registers have been collecting data. The 10-year CRR because of infection for patients having a primary hip arthroplasty in 1995 was 0.5% but for those operated in 1979 it was 1.2%. The 10-year CRR because of infection for OA patients operated with total knee arthroplasty during the years 1996–2000 was 1.0% but for those operated during 1976–1980 is was 4% (■ Fig. 3.4a). Rheumatoid patients have had a 2 times higher CRR rate because of infection than OA patients (■ Fig. 3.4b) with the exception of the cohort of patients operated after the year 2000 which does not have significantly higher CRR. The CRR for OA patients receiving a unicompartmental knee arthroplasty is lower than for those receiving a total knee arthroplasty (■ Fig. 3.4c). Men have higher CRR because of infection than women.

The majority of the infections arise early. Awareness in the early post-operative period in-

■ **Table 3.1.** The number of primary hip and knee arthroplasties revised for the first time during 2003–2007 because of infection

Year	Hip	Knee	Total
2003	90	55	145
2004	82	53	135
2005	85	65	150
2006	80	61	141
2007	104	65	169
Total	441	299	740

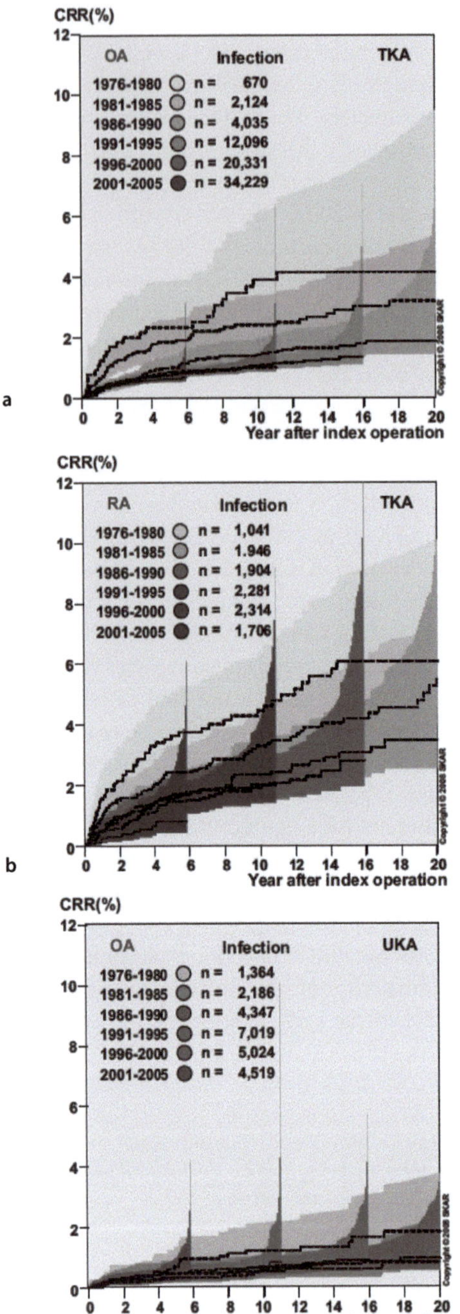

Fig. 3.4a–c. The 10 year cumulative revision rate (CRR) because of infection for patients; **a** with osteoarthritis (OA) primary operated with total knee arthroplasty (TKA), **b** with rheumatoid arthritis (RA) primary operated with TKA and **c** with OA primary operated with unicompartmental knee arthroplasty (UKA). (Published with permission from the Swedish knee arthroplasty register)

creases the likelihood of early detection and thereby the possibility to treat the infection with retention of the implant (Zimmerli et al. 1998). One of the variables reported by the hip arthroplasty register is re-operation within 2 years, where not only true revisions with exchange or removal of implants are included but even soft tissue operations. 0.6% of primary hip arthroplasties performed from 2004 to 2007 were re-operated within 2 years because of infection. This variable is officially published for every department and there was a variation between departments from 0% to 2.8%.

The infecting organism is not registered in the individual case but the microbiology has been studied in research projects (Ostendorf et al. 2004). In a study on 960 first-time revisions of hip arthroplasty due to infection during 1979 to 2000 information about the infecting pathogen was available in 573 cases. Coagulase-negative Staphylococcus was the most common cause of infection, accounting for 36.1% of the infections, followed by Staphylococcus aureus which accounted for 18.7%. Streptococcus species accounted for 8.6%, other gram-positive bacteria for 8.4%, gram-negative bacteria 9.9%, anaerobic bacteria 7.7% and in 10.8% there was a mixed culture with more than one infecting pathogen. Throughout the period there was a proportional increase in the number of infections caused by coagulase-negative Staphylococcus and a decrease in the number of infections caused by gram-negative bacteria. Methicillin-resistant Staphylococcus aureus have caused some cases of infected hip- and knee arthroplasty in Sweden but to date the efforts taken to keep MRSA out of hospitals have been successful. The coagulase-negative Staphylococcus has become increasingly resistant to methicillin and now approximately 70% of isolates at hospitals are methicillin-resistant.

The most common type of treatment has been two-stage revision. In a study on 960 first-time revisions of hip arthroplasty due to infection from 1979 to 2000 (Ostendorf et al. 2004) 56.2% were treated by two-stage revision, 26.9% were treated by one-stage revision and 16.9% with permanent extraction of the prosthesis. Two-stage revision is the dominating type of treating infected knee arthroplasties, followed by primary arthrodesis.

Discussion

The true infection rate after primary hip- and knee arthroplasty is not known. The registers report the cumulative revision rate which reflects the infection rate but can be influenced by how active the orthopaedic surgeons are in their efforts to diagnose and surgically treat infection. Without clear definition of infection and without standardised ways of measuring infection rate, comparison is difficult. No other national register provides information on the true infection rate. What can be compared is the number of revisions because of infection in relation to the number or primary arthroplasties, and when doing this it seems that the burden of infection in Sweden is comparable to or lower than reported by other registers (Norwegian Arthroplasty Register 2008; Australian Orthopedic Association 2008; National Joint Registry for England and Wales).

The cumulative infection rate was much higher during the first years of the registers and the prophylactic measures developed have had an effect (Lidgren 2001). It is however uncertain if the infection rate can be lowered further and there are concerns about the future that are related to development of resistant bacterial strains, larger number of frail and immunologically compromised patient having an arthroplasty and increased load in the healthcare system with risk of reluctance with respect to prophylactic routines. In a survey recently done by the knee register it was found that the administration of the systemic antibiotic prophylaxis in half of the cases was suboptimal (unpublished material from the Swedish knee arthroplasty register). Continuous efforts are needed to ensure that prophylactic routines are followed, both with regard of antibiotics but even other prophylactic measures. Increased knowledge on the pathophysiology of foreign body infection will hopefully add to the options available for the prevention and treatment of infection in the future.

There is a trend towards more open access to department-specific register data and even ranking of departments. The aim of open comparison is to encourage local improvement and there are good examples about departments reacting properly to reduce problems identified and published by the registers. Several problems have however been pointed out when interpreting the results and awareness of those problems is of utmost importance. It is difficult if not impossible to adjust for differences in case-mix or change the fact that the results are historical (Robertsson et al. 2006). There are risks with ranking of hospitals based on reported complications. Correct interpretation is necessary to avoid conclusions based on ranking lists without consideration of spuriously occurring data scatter. Recently, specific statistical methods to calculate the confidence interval of the ranking have been suggested to address this problem (Ranstam et al. 2008).

Conclusion

The Swedish arthroplasty registers are well established, with national coverage and reliable methods of registration. Swedish orthopaedic surgeons are using relatively few types of implants and even though the use of carefully chosen uncemented hip implants has increased, cementing technique is dominating. Principally, all cement used contains gentamicin and the most common systemic antibiotic prophylaxis is cloxacillin. The 10-year CRR because of infection is low, 0.5% for primary hip arthroplasty and 1.0% for primary knee arthroplasty, but due to the increasing number of arthroplasties the burden of infection increases. Continuing efforts are needed to keep down the infection rate and there is a need for research to evaluate and develop prophylactic measures.

References

Australian Orthopedic Association (2008) Hip and Knee Arthroplasty, annual report 2008. Available at www.dmac.adelaide.edu.au/aoanjrr

Kärrholm J, Garellick G, Herberts P (2007) Swedish hip arthroplasty register, annual report 2007. Available at http://www.jru.orthop.gu.se

Lidgren L (2001) Joint prosthetic infections: A success story. Acta Orthop Scand 72: 553–555

National Joint Registry for England and Wales. 4th Annual Report. Available at www.njrcentre.org.uk

Ostendorf M, Eisler T, Herberts P, Fleer A, van der Tweel I, Dhert WJA, Malchau H (2004) Results after revision THA because of deep infection. Trends and risk factors in 960 first revisions in the Swedish National Hip Registry. Thesis, Utrecht

Ranstam J, Wagner P, Robertsson O, Lidgren L (2008) Healthcare quality registers: outcome-orientated ranking of hospitals is unreliable. J Bone Joint Surg Br 90: 1558–1561

Robertsson O, Dunbar M, Knutson K, Lewold S, Lidgren L (1999) Validation of the Swedish Knee Arthroplasty Register. A postal survey regarding 30,376 knees operated on between 1975 and 1995. Acta Orthop Scand 70: 462–472

Robertsson O, Lewold S, Knutson K, Lidgren L (2000) The Swedish Knee Arthroplasty Project. Acta Orthop Scand 71: 7–18

Robertsson O, Lidgren L (2008) Annual report 2008, The Swedish Knee Arthroplasty Register. Available at http://www.knee.se

Robertsson O, Ranstam J, Lidgren L (2006) Variation in outcome and ranking of hospitals: an analysis from the Swedish knee arthroplasty register. Acta Orthop 77: 487–493

The Norwegian Arthroplasty Register (2008) Report 2008. Available at www.haukeland.no/nrl

Zimmerli W, Widmer AF, Blatter M, Ochsner PE (1998) Role of rifampicin for treatment of orthopedic implantrelated staphylococcal infections. JAMA 279: 1537–1541

Status and Prospect of an European Arthroplasty Register (EAR)

Sebastian Gaiser

Introduction

Arthroplasty Registers deliver important outcomes research parameters (Patt and Mauerhan 2005). The main indicators are implant survival and revision rates. Registers are established on a national or regional level. International comparison of registers is a challenge as the registration and the publication of results differ (Labek et al. 2008). From international prognosis it is obvious that knee and hip incidence will further increase and will remain a medical and economic burden to societies (Fig. 4.1; Kim 2008). Therefore outcomes research in the field of arthroplasty will help medical personal and decision makers in the healthcare market to base their decisions on relevant evidence.

EAR (European Arthroplasty Register) longs for a collaboration of the National Arthroplasty Registers in Europe to improve comparability of data and wants to serve as an international warning system for implant failure. EAR is consulting and supporting the establishment of new arthroplasty registers.

The establishment of a German register and the commitment of industry to establish a valid implant database for registers is a first step which may help to harmonize data. Bringing national and regional registers together for joint research and exchange of information will most likely resume to happen on a project based approach. Harmonizing data creation and publication will remain a challenge for EAR. Currently EAR is the platform in Europe to enhance the exchange of information between registers. Based on presentations by EAR and research by national registers the following prospects for EAR can be considered.

Possible Prospects for EAR and International Approaches to Arthroplasty Registers

Online Solution to Bring Together Research Findings and Proposals for Collaborative, Interdisciplinary and Multi-Register Studies

Registers like the Swedish National Hip Arthroplasty Register can closely work with other patient-related information such as patient-reported outcome measurements and even other National Registers as installed in Sweden (Weimin 2009). Therefore, research findings often go beyond the usual implant related topics. Recent findings were published on the increased risk of obese patients to acquire an acute infection after primary hip arthroplasty (Dowsey and Choong 2008a,b) and

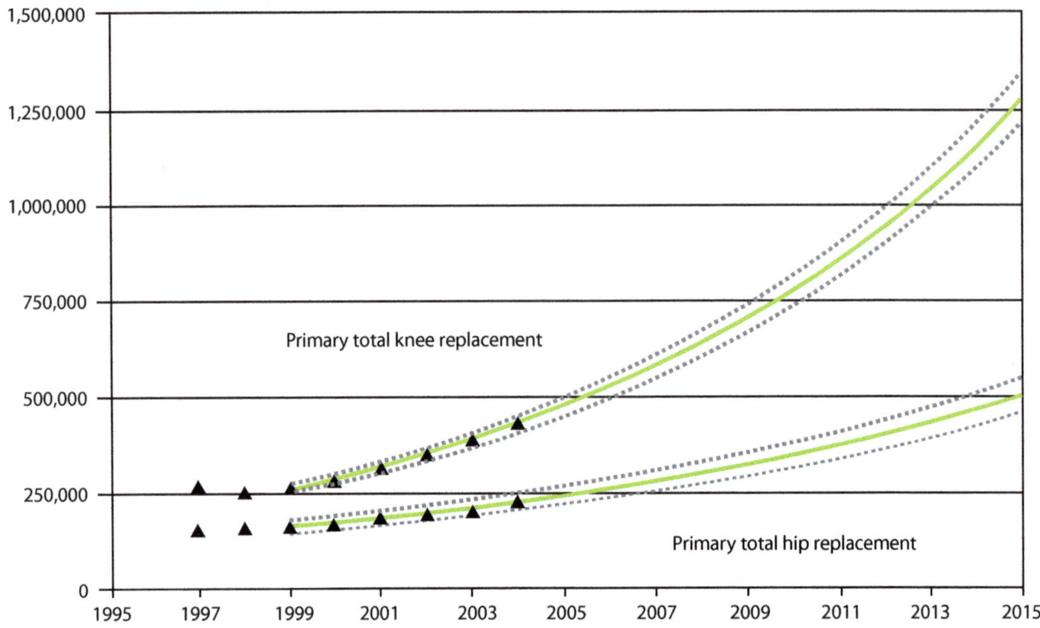

Fig. 4.1. Prognosis of total hip- and knee replacement in the USA up to 2015 (From: Kim 2008)

taking into account patient-reported outcomes such as the pre-operative EQ-5D anxiety/depression dimension which was a strong predictor for pain relief and patient satisfaction after surgery (Rolfson et al. 2009). These topics, even though researched in a specific population, may be of interest to closely watch in other register populations as they may help further identify outcome-related causes. EAR could establish an online solution to bring together research findings and proposals for collaborative, interdisciplinary and multi-register studies.

Humans Resources: Learning Curve, Training and Surgeon Shortage

Learning-curve explanations are often raised in the context of differences in register outcomes for established products, operating method or use of new technology (Cobb et al. 2007). International learning-curve findings can be addressed through a platform such as EAR to ensure appropriate training options and may help to develop helpful guidelines for technologies with well-understood evidence for good outcomes but poor adoption. Education on registers is still poor in some European countries and attendance of orthopaedic surgeons at e.g. EFORT meetings has room for improvement. Surgeon shortage is or will become of concern to many countries as prognosed demographic changes in incidence become reality (Kim 2008; Comeau 2004; Kurtz et al. 2007).

Registers – Determine a Way to Finance It

Any concept of a new register faces the challenge to determine a way to finance it. Several different models have been applied in European countries (Kolling et al. 2007). Questions remain: What kind of model can set the appropriate incentives for doctors, hospitals, sickness funds, private insurance companies and industry to serve the intentions of a register best? What are the actual costs and benefits of establishing and running a register? These questions will be important to assess in the future. First input can be expected from the DIMDI (Deutsches Institut für Medizinische Dokumentation und Information) HTA Report on arthroplasty registers which incorporates juridical, ethical, social, and »cost-efficiency« aspects (DIMDI 2009). Further longitudinal health economic assessments are necessary to make the medical and financial impacts transparent to countries which have no registers yet.

Industry Product Database

The German implant and bone cement industry organized under BVMed (Bundesverband Medizintechnologie e.V.) has announced that it is willing to finance the establishment of a German product database of implants and bone cements for the German register (BVMed 2009). This database can serve as an important milestone in consolidating the database of all established and new registers. Therefore, industry could register all products sold and implanted in European countries. In case this database is available to all registers, it will ease and support the creation of new registers in and outside Europe as one of the first hurdles is already taken. Industry commitment to such a database is also a step to improve the transparency of interactions between industry, researchers and users. The need for improved quality assurance resp. a German Arthroplasty Register has been discussed since the early 1980s (Schmid 1984).

Conclusion

Any multinational institution such as EAR dealing with arthroplasty registers has several options of topics which they can cover: The need to prioritize will be a major task of any institution in this field. The role of patients, sickness funds, private health insurers and industry needs to be addressed to increase the visibility and importance of national registers. EAR's network can only grow and sustain if financing is ensured. The opportunity of EAR for the EFORT organization is significant: However participation of orthopaedic surgeons in register-focused sessions during congresses has been fairly low. Bringing together all research and outcomes on one platform will be a helpful tool to further improve treatment and decrease overall costs of arthroplasty.

References

BVMed (2009) Qualitätssicherung bei Gelenkersatz: BVMed-Hersteller sagen G-BA Beteiligung am Endoprothesenregister zu. Online Source

Cobb JP, Kannan V, Brust K, Thevendran G (2007) Navigation reduces the learning curve in resurfacing total hip arthroplasty. Clin Orthop Relat Res 463: 90–97

Comeau P (2004) Crisis in orthopedic care: surgeon and resource shortage. CMAJ 171: 223

DIMDI (2009) Was sind die medizinischen Vor- und Nachteile von Endoprotheseregistern? Welche internationalen Erfahrungen gibt es? Wie sieht es mit der Kosteneffektivität aus? Welche juristischen, ethischen und sozialen Aspekte spielen mit ein? Available at http://www.dimdi.de/static/de/hta/programm/prioritaeten.htm

Dowsey MM, Choong PF (2008) Early outcomes and complications following joint arthroplasty in obese patients: a review of the published reports. ANZ J Surg 78: 439–444

Dowsey MM, Choong PF (2008) Obesity is a major risk factor for prosthetic infection after primary hip arthroplasty. Clin Orthop Relat Res 466: 153–158

Kim S (2008) Changes in surgical loads and economic burden of hip and knee replacements in the US: 1997–2004. Arthritis Rheum 59: 481–488

Kolling C, Simmen BR, Labek G, Goldhahn J (2007) Key factors for a successful National Arthroplasty Register. J Bone Joint Surg Br 89: 1567-1573

Kurtz SM, Ong KL, Schmier J et al. (2007) Future clinical and economic impact of revision total hip and knee arthroplasty. J Bone Joint Surg Am 89 (Suppl 3): 144–151

Labek G, Stoica CI, Bohler N (2008) Comparison of the information in arthroplasty registers from different countries. J Bone Joint Surg Br 90: 288–291

Patt JC, Mauerhan DR (2005) Outcomes research in total joint replacement: a critical review and commentary. Am J Orthop 34: 167–172

Rolfson O, Dahlberg LE, Nilsson JA, Malchau H, Garellick G (2009) Variables determining outcome in total hip replacement surgery. J Bone Joint Surg Br 91: 157–161

Schmid O (1984) Genaue Dokumentation erforderlich - Qualitätssicherung bei Gelenkimplantaten. Niedersächsisches Ärzteblatt 23/1984

Weimin YE (2009) Swedish Health Register. Online Source

The Infected Implant – Microbiology and Clinical Strategies

Ian Stockley

Sepsis after total joint arthroplasty is a devastating complication resulting in significant morbidity for the patient and adversely affecting prosthetic outcome. The advent of antibiotic prophylaxis, clean air enclosures and improved patient selection have all contributed to a decrease in the incidence of deep infection but with the increasing number of arthroplasties being performed, the prevalence of deep infection has increased.

Pathophysiology of Joint Infections

All surgical wounds are contaminated by bacteria and as Lord Moynihan said »every surgical procedure is an experiment in bacteriology«. Infection will become established when the dose of bacteria with its inherent virulence overcomes host defences. It is difficult to say why some patients become infected and others do not, considering the degree of bacterial contamination identified at surgery. It seems safe to assume that, as well as surgical and environmental factors, patient factors e.g. Immune factors play an important role in the development of clinical infection. Bacteria approach the surface of prosthesis through an interaction of physical and chemical forces. Host proteins promote attachment of bacteria onto the implant. Adhesion progresses to aggregation of bacteria on the surface of the prosthesis where they become encased in a matrix of polysaccharides and proteins to form a slimy layer known as a biofilm. Bacteria in the biofilms grow slowly and can resist cellular and humoral immune responses. In addition, they are much more resistant to antibiotics than when they are in their planktonic phase. MICs often elevated to a 1000 fold. Biofilm inhibition using quorum sensing inhibitor RIP is an exciting new area and may well change the management of prosthetic joint infection until then biomaterial-related infections will, in general, not clear until the implant is removed and antibiotics are given.

Management of Prosthetic Joint Infection

Most prosthetic joint infections are chronic infections by the time of clinical presentation. Acute infections i.e. early postoperative and haematogenous infections are relatively rare. The sooner they are diagnosed and treated accordingly, the better the results. Unfortunately diagnosis and referral are often delayed. Diagnosis after 3 weeks has a success rate of prosthesis retention, of less than 10%. If picked up within 1 week then the success rate climbs to 70%. Debridement of the joint followed by aggressive antibiotic therapy is the treatment of choice.

The management of chronic infection is primarily surgical with antibiotics having a supporting role only. Exchange arthroplasty offers the best results with respect to postoperative function. The surgical decision is whether to offer surgery as a direct exchange procedure or in a two-staged fashion. Control of infection results tends to be better when a two-stage regime is undertaken. However, it needs to be noted that this involves two major surgical procedures along with associated morbidities with costs to both the patient and the hospital institution. There are many treatment variables with the two-stage procedure including: length of the interval between the two stages, antibiotic policy and the choice of implants used for reconstruction, thus making comparison of results from different centres difficult. Antibiotics can be given systemically or delivered locally by antibiotic-loaded cement beads or cement spacers. Local delivery systems have the advantage of high local concentrations being eluted at the site and so have maximum therapeutic effect on the damaged infected tissues. The use of cement spacers eluting antibiotic is very attractive as this has the added benefits of allowing the patient to mobilise between the stages and also lessens the degree of shortening resulting from scar. Prolonged courses of intravenous antibiotic have been proposed by many authors, but recent work suggests that this may not be necessary if appropriate antibiotic is added to the cement at both the first and second stages.

Cementless reconstructive techniques are becoming increasingly popular and the concept of antimicrobial coatings on the prosthesis may even allow for these prostheses to be used in a single stage procedure in the future.

It is evident that not all infections behave in the same way and surgeons do differ in their approach to the management of the patient with an infected arthroplasty. A treatment regime offering the best possible outcome for each individual patient should be selected accordingly. Whilst surgery plays a major role in the management of these cases, interaction and discussion with a dedicated microbiologist is essential for success.

Infection of Joint Prosthesis and Local Drug Delivery

Andrzeij Górecki, Ireneusz Babiak

Introduction

The rapidly raising number of joint arthroplasties performed around the world yearly is accompanied by the certain percentage of different complications. The infection of the implant is one of the most important clinically, both for the patient and for the treating center. The problem of diagnosis and treatment of the postoperative infection is well known, but there is still lack of optimal, precise guidelines for medical action. Different centers developed their own strategies. Many experimental and clinical trials have been already performed to improve the results of treatment and still many promising concepts and methods are under investigation. Many conferences are organized and many materials are published to enable doctors to exchange their experience in fighting the problem (Langlais 2003; Buchholz et al. 1981).

Prevalence, Nature and Consequences of Periprosthetic Infection

Periprosthetic infection is a rare complication of the most frequent orthopaedic operation. It can lead to severe consequences like destruction of the bone stock and failure of the arthroplasty including amputation or even death of the patient due to general sepsis. Despite its low percentage, the direct number of infected prostheses increases every year due to improved survival of modern implants and due to increased lifetime of patients with implanted prostheses who are at risk of late and hematogenous infection, which are the dominant forms of infection (Ainscow and Denham 1984; Estrada et al. 1994; Widmer 2001).

The exact prevalence of infection complicating arthroplasty is an open issue. It depends on criteria which are used for recognition, the reliability of different diagnostic tools and follow-up of patients. The published data seems to be a little confusing, as there is not sure if published percentage regards only to the first year after arthroplasty, or includes cumulative number of every case of late or hematogenous infection which manifests even two decades after the operation. The infection after primary arthroplasty occurs in 0,5–1% cases of total hip, 0,5–2% of total knee, about 1% of total shoulder, 5,3–11% of total elbow, 3,1% of total ankle replacements and 2–8% of spinal fusions. On the other hand, infection can be the reason of 5–12% revisions. If diagnosis is based on non-culture techniques like PCR or fluorescence scanning microscopy, the reported incidence of infections is higher comparing to the cultures alone (Estrada et al. 1994; Lonner et al. 1996; Tunney et al. 1999; Zimmerli et al. 2004). At our department a special septic unit was created for treatment of musculoskeletal infections, and many patients are referred from other hospitals for therapy. Our own statistics shows, that during the decade 1994–2003 early infections constituted 25%, late and after revisions 69% and hematogenous 6% from totally 112 treated septic hip prostheses (Babiak and Górecki 2002).

Costs of therapy of a single-infected prosthesis differ between national medical care systems. For example, one infected case of hip prosthesis in the USA in the year 2000 »costs« 60,000–75,000 $. Similar costs in Germany (in 2003) were 50,000 EU per case, in Great Britain (2003) 75,000 EU and total costs in Great Britain were 170 million EU. Total expenses for therapy of infected arthroplasties can consume 7% of budget of university hospital (Gaston 2007; Loraas and Skrami 2004; Sculco 1995).

The development of implant infection is based on biofilm formation including the quorum-sensing mechanism of cooperation between microorganisms. The plurality and differentiation of bacteria from planctonic into sessile forms in mature biofilm emerges resistance of bacteria against antibiotics. The doses of antibiotics active in vitro against planctonic forms of bacteria, in biofilm conditions can require 200–1000 folds higher concentrations of the same drug. In consequence, it makes it impossible to cure active periprosthetic infection by means of systemic antibiotics which in doses active in biofilm can be toxic for patient when used systematically (Balaban et al. 2005; Costeron 2005).

Diagnosis and Therapy of Periprosthetic Infection

The recognition of periprosthetic infection is based on clinical, microbiological and histological criteria. It is easy to diagnose early infection whereas late infection can give non-specific symptoms, and thus can be recognised at the stage of septic loosening (Estrada et al. 1994; Mangram et al. 1999). Despite of number of publications and activity of two major scientific societies dealing with this problem there is still lack of EBM supported clear guidelines for therapy of infected prosthesis. It may be

partially due to the lack of control group – treated without systemic antibiotics in the antibiotic era. Current practice in many countries in case of early infection includes surgical debridement, i.e. excision of infected tissue layer surrounding implant, »diluting« lavage with copious volume of sterile saline solution, brushing, sonication of implant or tissue surface, exchange of all mobile components of prosthesis, application of local antimicrobials and postoperative systemic antimicrobial therapy (Buchholz et al. 1981; Babiak and Górecki 2002; Gaston 2007; Lidwell 1982; Malizos et al. 2007; Zimmerli et al. 2004).

More differences are noted between health care systems and different countries in case of late and hematogenous infection. Up to date there is an agreement as to general rules of treatment and details depend on anatomic location of infected prosthesis:

1. Permanent removal of prosthesis
2. Two-stage replacement
3. One-stage replacement
4. Arthrodesis
5. Amputation
6. Suppressive antimicrobial chemotherapy

Mean infection control rates under different therapy protocols of infected THR which can be find in publications are listed in order of increasing success rate (Callaghan et al. 1999; Lidwell 1982; Zimmerli et al. 2004; Babiak and Górecki 2002; Buttaro et al. 2005; Witso and Engesaeter 2007):

- 58% – one-stage replacement using cement without antibiotic,
- 60–86% – only suppressive antibiotic therapy (results in the course of therapy),
- 82% – two-stage replacement using cement without antibiotic,
- 83% – one-stage replacement using cement with antibiotic,
- 88% – Girdlestone procedure (permanent removal of prosthesis),
- 89,9% – cementless reimplantation – one- or two-stage,
- 91% – two-stage replacement – cement with antibiotic,
- 93–97% – two-stage reimplantation – cemented with allogenic bone grafts.

Local Antibiotic Delivery Systems

Since the periprosthetic infection occurs mainly in tissues surrounding directly prosthesis surface, local delivery of antimicrobial agent is now and seems to be in the future the choice option in therapy and prophylaxis of implant infection. From historical point of view, the local antimicrobial therapy preceeded systemic treatment. In 1892 Dressman first used plaster of Paris (calcium sulfate) with antiseptic substances. In 1928 Petrova added 10% rivanol to plaster of Paris. In 1947 DeGrood applicated bone graft with penicillin. In the 1960s polyglycolid acid (PGA) and polylactid acid (PLA) were introduced in form of sheets. In the 1970s Buchholz and Klemm started the usage of antibiotic-loaded acrylic cement. In the 1980s natural polymers gained form of pins and pellets which were more suitable for orthopedic surgery, and in 1982 Buri and Lob promoted *Taurolin gel.* In 1987 Ascherl and Stemberger introduced *Garamycin Schwamm.* Since 1989, gentamicin and fucidin was added to pellets. In the 1990s bone graft with antibiotics gained clinical importance as local antimicrobial therapy. Every year an increasing number of natural and synthetic material is tested and introduced as carriers of antibiotics (Hanssen 2005; Klem 1993; Stemberger et al. 2007; Walenkamp 1997).

The ideal antimicrobial agent should provide high local concentration without systemic toxicity of the drug, should be active against sessile form of bacteria and should not impair bone regeneration and biologic incorporation of implant. The osteoinductive and osteoconductive properties are also desired. Local antibiotic concentrations reported in literature are 3800–4746 ug/ml (Hanssen 2005). Higher concentrations are potentially nephrotoxic. Despite the wide usage of local antimicrobial therapy there are still open questions regarding optimal and maximal local concentration of the drug, the necessity for therapeutic effect longevity of antimicrobial activity and the influence of antimicrobials on bone regeneration. Some drugs like quinolones, gentamicin and rifamicin have already known dose-dependent inhibition effect on bone reparation (Hanssen 2005; Witso and Engesaeter 2007; Trampuz and Zimmerli 2006).

Currently used local drug delivery vehicles are grossly divided into resorbable and non-resorbable ones. The first drug-delivery system provide high initial local doses with decrease of antibiotic concentration in the course of degradation of a carrier.

Local drug delivery carriers used in musculoskeletal infections:
1. Bone cements
2. Bone grafts
3. Bone graft substitutes or extenders
4. Natural polymers
5. Synthetic polymers
6. Composite biomaterials

Non-absorbable carriers ensure initially therapeutic concentration of drug which is followed by sustained level of antibiotic for longer time. Recently new drug delivery systems are developed, which in the way of intermittent pulsing allow to achieve high doses of antibiotic, thus allowing attack of sessile bacteria that have become planctonic. As regards physicochemical properties local antibiotic delivery systems for therapy of osteomyelitis and orthopaedic device-related infections include now six classes of carriers (Hanssen 2005).

1. **Antibiotic-loaded acrylic bone cements** (ALBC, ALAC) are today regarded as gold standard (Blaha et al. 1993; Evans and Nelson 1993; Klem 1993; Walenkamp 2007). It is necessary to differ between acrylic cement containing low dose and high dose of antibiotic. Low-dose ALACs contain mostly less than 1 g of aminoglycosides, colistin or erythromycin per 40 g of polymer and are widely used as prophylactic measure in primary arthroplasty. There are statistical data pointing that application of low-dose ALAC allowed to reduce 11-fold the incidence of septic complications after THR (Lidwell 1982). But early studies in animals did not prove expectation regarding the protective role of gentamicin-loaded cement against hematogenous infection (Blomgren and Lindgren 1981). High-dose ALAC plays the role mainly in revisions of infected prostheses – as material for spacer formation and for insertion of a new prosthesis at 2nd stage or during one-stage replacement. It can be also used for staged seg-

mental bone-defect reconstruction for example in Masquelet procedure (Pelissier et al. 2004). The use of ALAC spacers in septic THR revision was started by Duncan in 1993 (Duncan and Beauchamp 1993). Now, depending on the experience or preferred option by treating surgeon, the hand-made or prefabricated spacers can be used. The role of this temporary implant is local delivery of antibiotic, avoidance of dead-space formation and preventing of soft-tissue contraction. There are two types of spacers: first generation – static spacers – and second generation – articulated spacers. The term PROSTALAC is an acronym for PROSTthesis of Antibiotic-Loaded Acrylic Cement. The antibiotic remains in ALAC in form of inclusions and in this way gives the ALAC-porous structure. This allows elution of antibiotic from ALAC which takes place from the outer surface of cement. The acrylic cement containing 5% of antibiotics fulfils ISO standard regarding resistance against compressive forces (minimum 70 mPa; respective with 5% of vancomycin – 95 mPa). Optimal, experimentally stated content of antibiotic in cement for inserting prosthesis varies between 2,5 and 7,5% with a maximum of 10% for temporary spacer. It was experimentally established in animal models that gentamicin may diffuse from ALAC to adjacent bone in concentrations 4-folds higher than MIC for more than 6 months (Langlais 2004). In an other experiment it was stated that at an average 20% of all admixed antibiotic is eluted after implantation of spacer and that 15% of antibiotic is eluted from ALAC during 2 weeks after implantation. When low-dose gentamicin-loaded cement is used for implantation of prosthesis, periprosthetic haematoma after THR can contain antibiotic in concentration 20-folds over MIC (Langlais 2004). Aminoglycosides, vancomycin, teicoplanin, cefalosporines, clindamycin, colistin, ciprofloxacin, meropenem are recommended for mixing with acrylic cement, whereas penicillines, lincomycin, chloramphenicol, tetracyclines, rifampicyn should not be mixed with acrylic cement (Haddad et al. 1999). Elution has a better profile when selected ATB is intraoperatively added to acrylic cement which is already loaded with any antibiotic by manufacturer. Despite advantages of ALAC there are few reports on toxic serum level of gentamicin eluted from ALAC (van Raaij et al. 2002).

2. **Bone grafts** as auto- or allografts were primary used for filling the dead space after sequestrectomy. The advantage of bone graft is the combination of their osteoconductive properties with local release of antibiotic without evidence of toxicity (Witso et al. 2004). Antibiotics can be added in form of powder to morselised cancellous bone or the bone graft is soaked in antibiotic-containing solution (Witso and Engesaeter 2007; Winkler et al. 2000). Antibiotic is adsorbed on the surface of graft (◘ Fig. 6.1; Witso et al. 1999). Positive results of the use of vancomycin-, netilmicin- or tobramycin-soaked allograft in two-stage revisions have been clinically documented (Buttaro et al. 2005; Witso and Engesaeter 2007). In practical use, 1 g of vancomycin powder can be added to the morselised femoral head graft (Buttaro et al. 2005) and impacted into femur or acetabulum. Similiary safe and effective is the impregnation of 50 g of cancellous bone in solution containing 100 mg netilmicin per 1 ml (Witso and Engesaeter 2007). In such doses netilmicin and vancomycin do not impair incorporation of bone graft. In contrary, admixture of ciprofloxacin, gentamicin or rifamicin has a dose-dependent inhibition effect on bone reparation (Buttaro et al. 2005; Witso and Engesaeter 2007; Witso et al. 1999, 2004; Winkler et al. 2000).

3. **Bone graft substitutes or extenders** provide high local antibiotic concentration and simultaneously participate in the bone regeneration (◘ Fig. 6.2). Similar to bone graft, they can be used for filling of non-segmental bone defects which have form of voids and simultaneously for closure of dead space inside the bone. The advantage of substitutes is – in contrary to bone allografts – avoidance of pathogen transmission. Available products have form of pellets composed of calcium sulfate and 3.64% vancomycin (i.e. 1 g vancomycin per 25 g $CaSO_4$), calcium sulfate and 4,25% tobramicin (1.2 g tobramicin per 25 g $CaSO_4$), calcium hydroxya-

patite, calcium phosphates, bioactive glass, blood coated demineralised bone. It seems that due to their shape, diameter of pellets and quick resorption after implantation, this forms of bone-graft substitutes are not suitable to replace antibiotic impregnated morselised bone graft in septic revision of prosthesis (Hanssen 2005; Kawanabe et al. 1998; Lazarettos et al. 2004; Swieringa and Tulp 2005).

4. **Natural, protein-based polymers** use products derived from clotted blood or natural animal collagen for example antibiotic-loaded fibrin, thrombin or sponge collagen (Fig. 6.3; Hanssen 2005; Stemberger et al. 2007). They have the form of sheets and can be inserted after debridement in the early infection. Each form has its own elution profile of added antibiotic. After implantation of a collagen sponge containing 130 mg gentamicin, the therapeutic local level of gentamicin can maintain up to 5 days. It seems not to be safe to add antibiotic-containing polymers to one-stage revision with the use of high-dose antibiotic-loaded cement or together with ALAC spacer because of potential risk of

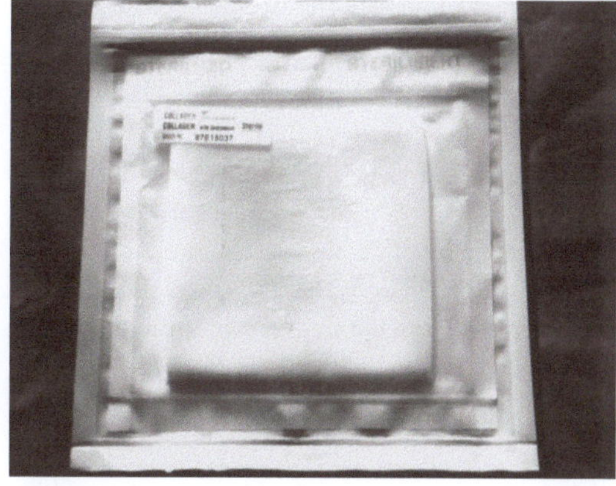

Fig. 6.1. Antibiotic-loaded bone graft

Fig. 6.3. Natural, protein-based polymers with ATB. (From Hanssen 2005)

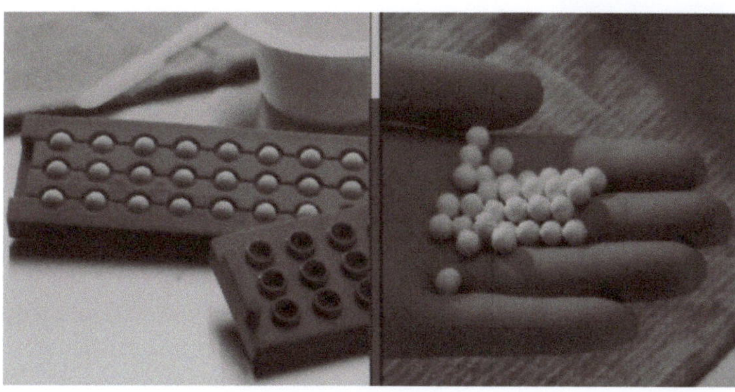

Fig. 6.2. Bone graft substitutes or extenders with ATB. (From Turner et al. 2005)

accumulation of antibiotic and its systemic toxic effect. Natural polymers have also the potential risk of transmission of prion-based diseases and allergic reactions, which were reported in 8% of patients. There are also reports on acute renal failure resulting from the toxic serum levels of gentamicin eluted from gentamicin collagen sponge (Swieringa and Tulp 2005).

5. **Synthetic polymers** represent resorbable, non-protein-derived carriers of antibiotics (Fig. 6.4). They enable to control and to adjust local antibiotic delivery during the time of degradation of the carrier. It is also possible to add other substances like growth factors. The polymers have the form of sheets, pins or disks. Because of the problem with their structural integrity, they are used mostly in the therapy of osteomyelitis. This class includes polymers like polyanhydrides, polylactid acid (PLA), polylactides-coglycolides (PLGA), polycaprolactone, cross-linked polydimethylsiloxane (PDMS). PLA and PLGA are in clinical use in orthopaedics (Hanssen 2005; Garvin and Feschuk 2005; Li et al. 2002; Nelson et al. 1997; Teupe et al. 1992).

6. **Composite biomaterials** have physicochemical characteristics necessary for osteoinduction and osteoconduction of the scaffold. They are able to provide delivery of antibiotic, participate in the bone regeneration and warrant structural integrity during the process of implant incorporation. They release antibiotics in different rates and time (Hanssen 2005). An example of composite biomaterial is hydroxyapatite scaffold drug-delivery system composed of polymeric foam with 87% porosity coated with a hybrid coating containing hydroxyapatite and antibiotic loaded polycapronate (Kim et al. 2004; Martins et al. 1998).

Prophylactic Measures Against Colonization and Development of Biofilm

Despite the established local antibiotic delivery systems including mostly different resorbable or nonresorbable vehicles – the non-cemented prosthesis and other cementless implants are at risk of late postoperative or hematogenous infection. For this implant or patients at higher risk of infection efforts must be made not only to cure diagnosed periprosthetic infection, but also to prevent development of postoperative infection. Currently practised or investigated measures for prevention of implant infections depend on fixation mode of joint prostheses. Low-dose antibiotic-loaded acrylic cement is now standard for cemented implants. For cementless implants many studies and trials are performed with coating of prosthesis with »cover« that becomes permeable for antimicrobial substance by low-frequency ultrasonic energy (»release on demand«), polymer layer forming carrier with incorporated antibiotic, porous hydroxyl apatite coatings containing antibiotic, coating with heavy metals (silver, copper) or heavy metal salts, coating with self-adhesive low-soluble antibiotic salts (Hanssen 2005; Kuhn and Vogt 2007). Other methods used or investigated independently of prosthesis fixation mode include inhibition of biofilm formation by quorum-sensing inhibitor RIP (RNA III inhibiting peptide; Balaban et al. 2005), increasing of gentamicin activity in biofilm by pulsed electromagnetic fields, increasing of vancomycin activity in biofilm by low-frequency ultrasound and modulation of non-specific immunological response by oral administration of phages after prosthesis revision in staphylococcal infection.

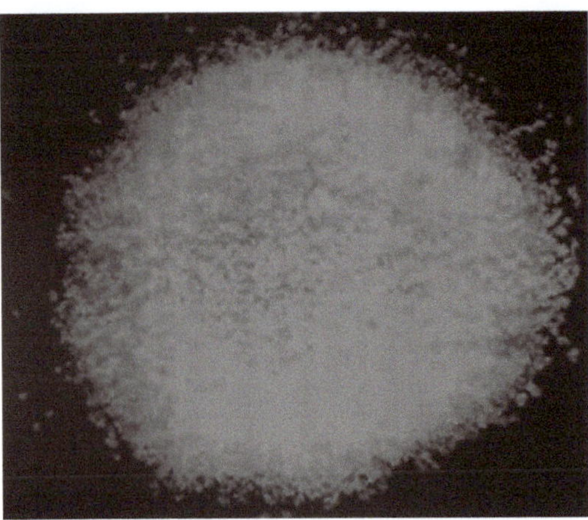

Fig. 6.4. Synthetic polymers with ATB (From Garvin and Feschuk 2005)

References

Ainscow DA, Denham RA (1981) The risk of hematogenous infection in total joint replacements. J Bone Joint Surg Br 66: 580–582

Babiak I, Górecki A (2002) Treatment outcome in infections complicating total hip replacements. Orthop Traumatol Rehab 4 (Suppl 1): 49–52

Balaban N, Stoodley P, Fux CA, Wilson S, Costerton JW, Dell'Acqua G (2005) Prevention of staphylococcal biofilm-associated infections by the quorum sensing inhibitor RIP. CORR 437: 48–54

Blaha JD, Calhoun JH, Nelson CL, Henry SL, Seligson D, Esterhai JL Jr, Heppenstall RB, Mader J, Evans RP, Wilkins J (1993) Comparison of the clinical efficacy and tolerance of gentamicin PMMA beads on surgical wire versus combined and systemic therapy for osteomyelitis. CORR 295: 8–12

Blomgren G, Lindgren U (1981) Late hematogenous infection in total joint replacement. Studies of gentamicin and bone cement in the rabbit. CORR 155: 244–248

Buchholz HW, Elson RA, Engelbrecht E, Lodenkaemper H, Roettger J, Siegel A (1981) Management of deep infection of total hip replacement. J Bone Joint Surg 63-B: 342–353

Buttaro M, Pusso R, Piccaluga F (2005) Vankomycin-supplemented impacted bone allografts in infected hip arthroplasty. Two-stage revision results. J Bone Joint Surg Br 87: 314–319

Callaghan JJ, Katz R., Johnston R (1999) One-stage revision surgery of the infected hip. Clin Orthop 369; 139–143

Costeron WJ (2005) Biofilm theory can guide the treatment of device related orthopaedic infections. CORR 437: 7–11

Duncan CP, Beauchamp C (1993) A temporary antibiotic-loaded joint replacement system for management of complex infections involving the hip. Orthop Clin North Am 24: 751–759

Estrada RR, Tsukayama D, Gustilo R (1994) Management of THA infections. A prospective study of 108 cases. Orthop Trans 17: 114–115

Evans RP, Nelson CL (1993) Gentamicin- impregnated polymethylmethacrylate beads compared with systemic antibiotic therapy in the treatment of chronic osteomyelitis. CORR 295: 37–42

Garvin K, Feschuk C (2005) Polylactide-polyglycolide Antibiotic Implants. 437: 105–110

Gaston P (2007) Diagnosis and management of infected arthroplasty – the United Kingdom experience. Local antibiotics in arthroplasty. Thieme, Stuttgart New York, pp 95–108

Haddad FS, Masri BA, Garbuz DS, Duncan CP (1999) The treatment of the infected hip replacement. CORR 369: 144–156

Hanssen A (2005) Local antibiotic delivery vehicles in the treatment of musculoskeletal infection. CORR 437: 91–96

Kawanabe K, Okada Y, Matsusue Y, Iida H, Nakamura T (1998) Treatment of osteomyelitis with antibiotic-soaked porous glass ceramic. J Bone Joint Surg 80(3): 527–530

Kim K, Luu YK, Chang C, Fang D, Hsiao BS, Chu B, Hadjiargyrou M (2004) Incorporation and controlled release of a hydrofilic antibiotic using poly(lactide-co-glycolide)-based electrospun nanofibrous scaffolds. J Control Release 98: 47–56

Klem WK (1993) Antibiotic bead chains. CORR 295: 63–76

Kuhn KD, Vogt S (2007) Antimicrobial implant coating in arthroplasty. Local antibiotics in arthroplasty. Thieme, Stuttgart New York, pp 23–29

Langlais F (2003) Can we improve the results of revision arthroplasty for infected total hip replacement? J Bone Joint Surg 85-B: 637–640

Langlais F (2004) Antibiotic cements in articular prostheses: current orthopaedic concepts. Int J Antimicrobial Agents 28: 84–89

Lazarettos J, Efstathopoulos N, Papagelopoulos PJ, Savvidou OD, Kanellakopoulou K, Giamarellou H, Giamarellos-Bourboulis EJ, Nikolaou V, Kapranou A, Papalois A, Papachristou G (2004) A bioresorbable calcium phosphate delivery system with teicoplanin for treating MRSA osteomyelitis. CORR 423: 253–258

Li LC, Deng J, Stephens D (2002) Polyanhydride implant for antibiotic delivery – from the bench to the clinic. Adv Drug Deliv Rev 54: 963–986

Lidwell L (1982) Effect of ultraclean air in operating rooms on deep sepsis in the joint after total hip or knee replacement: a randomised study. BMJ 10–14

Lonner JH, Desai P, Dicesare PE, Steiner G, Zuckerman JD (1996) The reliability of analysis of intraoperative frozen sections for identifying active infection during revision hip or knee arthroplasty. J Bone Joint Surg 78-B: 1553–1558

Loraas MV, Skrami IG (2004) Addend hospital expenses following re-admissions due to postoperative orthopaedic wound infections. Lecture 23nd Annual Meeting EBJIS Milano 27–29 May 2004

Malizos KN, Rodis NT (2007) Management of septic joint arthroplasty – the Hellenic experience. Local antibiotics in arthroplasty. Thieme, Stuttgart New York, pp 109–119

Mangram AJ, Horan TC, Pearson ML, Silver LC, Jarvis WR (1999) Guideline for prevention of surgical site infection. Centers for Disease Control and Prevention Hospital Infection Control Practices Advisory Committee. Am J Infect Control 27: 97–132

Martins VC, Goissis G et al. (1998) The controlled release of antibiotic by hydroxyapatite: anionic collagen composites. Artif Organs 22: 215–221

Nelson CL, Hickmon SG, Skinner RA (1997) Treatment of experimental osteomyelitis by surgical debridement and the implantation of biodegradable, polyanhydride-gentamicin beads. J Orthop Res 17: 249–255

Pelissier P, Masquelet AC, Bareille R, Pelissier SM, Amedee J (2004) Induced membranes secrete growth factors including vascular and osteoinductive factors and could stimulate bone regeneration. J Orthop Res 22: 73–79

Raaij van TM, Visser LE, Vulto AG, Verharr JA (2002) Acute renal failure after local gentamicin treatment in an infected total knee arthroplasty. J Arthroplasty 17: 948–950

Sculco TP (1995) The economic impact of infected total joint arthroplasty. Orthopaedics 18: 871–873

Stemberger A, Schwabe J, Ibrahim K, Matl F, Roessner M, Vogt S, Kühn KD (2007) New antibiotic carriers and coatings in surgery. Local antibiotics in arthroplasty. State of the art from an interdisciplinary point of view. Thieme, Stuttgart New York, pp 13–21

Swieringa AJ, Tulp NJ (2005) Toxic serum gentamicin levels after use of gentamicin -loaded sponges in in infected total hip arthroplasty. Acta Orthop 76: 75–77

Teupe C, Meffert R, Winckler S, Ritzerfeld W, Törmälä P, Burg E (1992) Ciprofloxacin-impregnated poly-L-lactic acid drug carrier; New aspects of a resorbable drug delivery system in local antimicrobial treatment of bone infections. Arch Orthop Trauma Surg 112: 33–35

Trampuz A, Zimmerli W (2006) Antimicrobial agents in orthopaedic surgery. Drugs 66: 1089–1105

Tunney MM, Patrick S, Curran MD, Ramage G, Hanna D, Nixon JR, Gorman SP, Davis RI, Anderson N (1999) Detection of prosthetic hip infection at revision arthroplasty by immunofluorescence microscopy and PCR amplification of the bacterial 16S rRNA gene. J Clin Microbiol 37: 3281–3290

Turner TM, Urban RM, Hall DJ, Chye PC, Segreti J, Gitelis S (2005) Local and systemic levels of tobramycin delivered from calcium sulfate bone graft substitute pellets. CORR 437: 97–104

Walenkamp GHIM (1997) Chronic osteomyelitis. Acta Orthop Scand 68: 497–506

Walenkamp GHIM (2007) Treatment of infected prostheses – the Dutch experience. Local antibiotics in arthroplasty. Thieme, Stuttgart New York, pp 133–143

Widmer AF (2001) New developments in diagnosis and treatment of infection in orthopedic implants. CID 33 (Suppl 2): 94–106

Winkler H, Janata O, Berger C, Wein W, Georgopoulos A (2000) In vitro release of vancomycin and tobramycin from impregnated human and bovine bone grafts. J Antimicrobial Chemot 46: 423–428

Witsø E, Persen L, Løseth K, Bergh K (1999) Adsorption and release of antibiotics from morselized cancellous bone. Acta Orthop Scand 70: 298–304

Witsø E, Persen L, Benum P, Aamodt A, Husby OS, Bergh K (2004) High local concentration without systemic adverse effects after impaction of netilmicin-impregnated bone. Acta Orthop Scand 75: 339–346

Witsø E, Engesaeter LB (2007) Revision of infected total hip prostheses in Norway and Sweden. Local antibiotics in arthroplasty. Thieme, Stuttgart New York, pp 145–146

Zimmerli W, Trampuz A, Ochsner PE (2004) Prosthetic joint infections. NEJM 351: 1645–1654

Clinical Strategy for the Treatment of Deep Infection of Hip Arthroplasty

David Jahoda

Since, the mid 1960s, the implantation of the arthroplasty has become the most popular orthopaedic operation and is one of the most successful therapeutical procedures performed by orthopaedic surgeons. Short-term success of the joint-replacement procedure produces excellent results. Patients once suffering from heavy pain, limping, markedly limited at work, social and sexual activities are suddenly completely cured. It is definitely not correct to underestimate the great effects of this procedure which, is a radical intervention into an organism. Almost 10% of the implanted joint replacements become complicated during its functioning. Most often, it is an aseptic loosening. Infectious complications are less frequent but far more devastating (Trampuz 2005).

There are many methods of treatment and although many of their propagators state 100% effectiveness, none of them are generally accepted as a method of choice. Preference of each method is given rather by rational problems, by region and history of the workplace.

It is clear that many of the methods are very successful in the hands of authors, but often they are transferred to another workplace in an incorrect way with worse results. Not only to copy the technique but to keep the ideological principle of the method is fundamental.

Failure of rifampicine which was glorified as a wonder drug for dissolving biofilm, in case of therapy without surgical intervention, is a typical example. It is proving unavoidable to match results by a modern manager routine like friendly benchmarking.

It is necessary to change this old strategy, when each workplace and region has its own favorite method which was promoted as the best one. We must admit that there are different types of patients, bacteria and kinds of infections with different diagnosis that delay and onset of the therapy.

Decisions of what kind of procedure will be used should be stated according to general status of the patient, type of agent and its glycocalix production and sensitivity to antibiotics. It is necessary to choose such a method that has in certain cases, the highest chance to eradicate the infection with the best possible functional result and at the same time the least challenging for the patient.

Individual approach concept for choosing the method of treatment was described by Zimmerli (◘ Fig. 7.1a,b; Zimmerli et al. 2004).

The surgical procedure is chosen according to type of infection, amount of symptoms, soft-tissue condition, stability of the implant and type of agent. We suppose that our scheme of using the PCR method in early diagnosis enables a much better way to set standards for the treatment process.

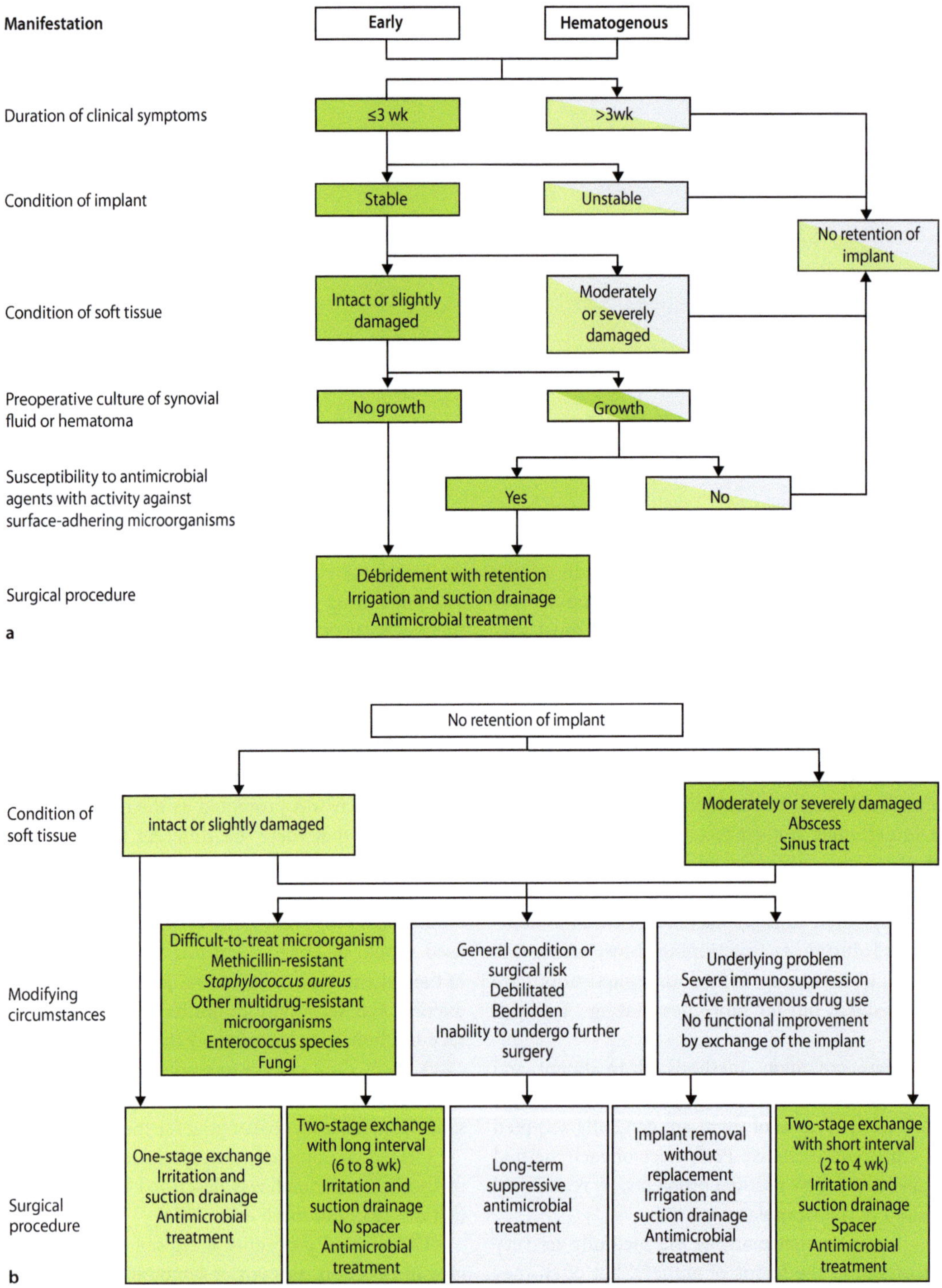

Manifestation

| Early | Hematogenous |

Duration of clinical symptoms — ≤3 wk / >3wk

Condition of implant — Stable / Unstable / No retention of implant

Condition of soft tissue — Intact or slightly damaged / Moderately or severely damaged

Preoperative culture of synovial fluid or hematoma — No growth / Growth

Susceptibility to antimicrobial agents with activity against surface-adhering microorganisms — Yes / No

Surgical procedure — Débridement with retention / Irrigation and suction drainage / Antimicrobial treatment

a

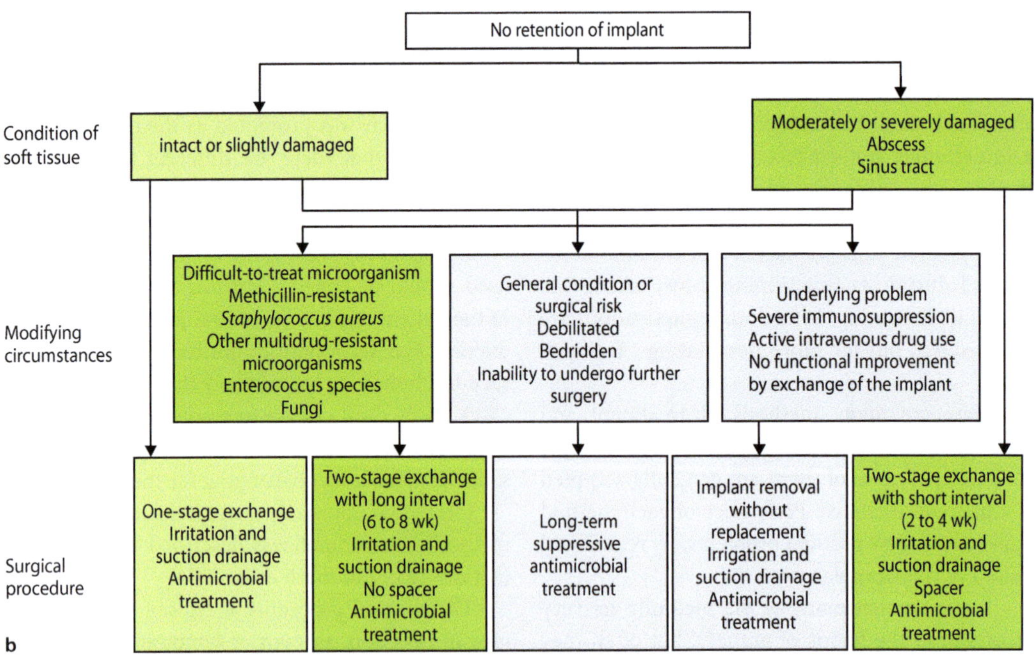

Fig. 7.1. a Algorithm for the treatment of early or hematogenous infection associated with a prosthetic joint by Zimmerli (2004). The surgical procedure is chosen according to the duration of symptoms, soft-tissue conditions, stability of the implants and type of agents. **b** Algorithm for the treatment of patients with infections not qualifying for implant retention by Zimmerli (2004). With this algorithm we can easily choice an optimal method for individual situations when we have to exchange implants

Table 7.1. New prognostic classification by Parvizi. This classification helps to determine the chances for success of treatment for single patients. Parvizi combined the Cireny classification with surgical factors and types of agent. The surgeon has the ability to provide better, more, and realistic patient information. Parvizi's classification will contribute to scientific comparisons (Parvizi et al. 2008)

	Class A	Class B	Class C
Host	Healthly (Cierny A, no comorbidity, no-smoker, well nutrished)	Moderate risk (Cierny B, some comorbidities, smoker, imperfect nutritional status)	Compromised (Cierny C, comorbidities, malnutrition, immunocompromised)
Surgical factors	Favorable (good soft tissues, minimal bone loss, early presentation)	Semi-compromised (late presentation, some soft tissue destruction, some bone loss)	Not favorable (soft-tissue destruction, bone loss, multiple surgeries, previous failures)
Organism	Favorable (pan-sensitive)	Semi-compromised (no organism, mild resistance)	Not favorable (resistant, multi-organism)
Success	80–100%	50–79%	Below 50%

Parvizi shows that individual approach is a current topic, he suggests new prognostic classification which enables us to better explain the advantages for the successful treatment to the patient (Table 7.1; Parvizi et al. 2008).

Timing is most important for the success of any treatment strategy. Setting of a diagnosis must be quick and correct. The keystone for setting the diagnosis must be the careful investigation of patient medical history and clinical examination. The meaning of this symptom is mentioned by some authors who set the diagnosis of an infection only on the basis of the presence of these signs (Vavřík et al. 2000).

If we evaluate changes in laboratory examinations, we can discover the increase of the leucocytes only in 15% of the patients with arthroplasty's deep wound infection. Sedimentation rate and C-reactive protein levels are the most commonly used and also most important lab exams for the evaluation of the infectious complications (Spangehl et al. 1997). At present, the blood level of CRP is becoming the most important and valued parameter (Santzen and Carlsson 1989). Although a low sedimentation rate does not exclude an infection of an arthroplasty as well.

X-ray pictures are a fundamental part of a diagnosis for a joint-replacement infection. Native X-rays are often normal within early stages of the infection. A radiolucent line which is usual in aseptic loosening can appear later. In the region of a hip joint a periostal reaction, quick migration of an implant and a diffuse osteolysis of a typical lacunary shape are typical signs of infection. We can find paraarticular ossifications in cases of mitigated infection. In the region of an endoprothetic stem we can find typical lacunary resorptions of a bubble shape (Fig. 7.2). Bony resorption in bone-cement interface is caused by an invasion of infected granulating tissue. Unfortunately these changes form after 3 to 6 months and that is why we cannot find them in cases of an early infection (Goldenberg 1989).

According to Tsukayama, classic three-phase scintigraphy with leucocytes marked by indium is very useful in diagnosing joint-replacement infection (Tsukayama et al. 2003).

Due to modern methods of detection, joint puncture is an examination which turns to be a gold standard for the diagnosis of infection. In the case of suspected joint-replacement deep infection, we perform puncture with precision keeping all aseptic guidelines, at best from mini-incision. Position of the needle should be verified by ultrasound, CT or arthrography (Widmer 2001). Incidence of false-negative results can be decreased by interruption of antibiotics two weeks before cultivation sampling, tapping (Barrack et al. 1997). It seems in our opinion to be an organization problem. Most

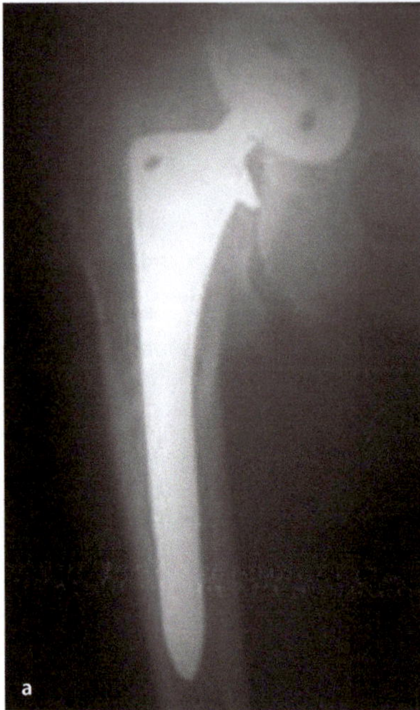
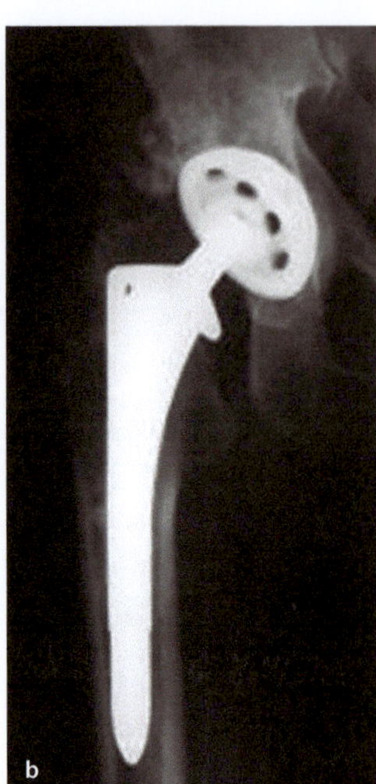

Fig. 7.2a,b. Acute hematogenic infection of the hip-joint replacement Duraloc/AML, successfully treated 2 weeds from the onset of the symptoms by revision, debridement, change of articulation surfaces and long-term antibiotic therapy by Drancourt scheme in 2001

of the patients already come with antibiotics from the general practitioner. Interruption of the antibiotics for two weeks extends the interval between beginning of the symptoms of infection and setting of the diagnosis, eventually surgical intervention. Protraction of this period decreases effect of the therapy of the infection (Vavřík et al. 2000; Jahoda et al. 2000). In our opinion we can reduce this interval by using PCR methods. Polymerase chain reaction (PCR) enables direct detection of the DNA of bacterial pathogens present in articulation fluid. By means of in-vitro multiplied DNA we detect the area of the genes that are typical for one bacterial species or the whole family. The principle of the PCR method is amplification chain reaction run by thermic alterations. Standard PCR detects DNA sequences and is suitable for demonstration of bacteria, candidas, and moulds. Quantitative PCR (qPCR) method is used for quantitative description of infection. Newly introduced »real-time« PCR significantly increases the attraction of molecular microbiological methods for us thanksfully for a higher pace, more correct quantification, lower risk of contamination, lower labor consumption and continuously raising reproduceability.

In certain applications the so-called »broad-range« PCR is used, detecting universal bacterial sequences. In case of broad-range PCR, the universal DNA primer (usually 16S ribosomal RNA genes), which is present in bacteria but not in humans or viruses, is used for amplification of DNA section. Results will be additionally compared with cultivation.

Our suggested scheme of using PCR in diagnosis of periprosthetic infection includes three steps. The first step is to detect by end-point PCR general presence of bacteria and fungi pathogenes in punctured substance with possible following specification by RFLP. In case of positive capture the second step will follow – examination of samples by multiplex PCR tested for the presence of the genes for ability to create biofilm and resistance to methicillin. In methicillin resistance there exist 5 types, and No. IV has 4 versions. The gene mecA was proved to be the most reliable for detection of the resistance to methicillin. As a third step the use of the multiplex PCR in real time detecting ability to create biofilm enables discrimination of S. aureus and S. epidermidis and detection of the virulence in Staphylococcus epidermidis.

Perioperative diagnosing does not offer us much chance to change the strategy. Only perioperative histology of frozen specimen could be useful. During the operation, frozen specimens could differentiate real infection from contamination. Accuracy of this technique depends on experience and knowledge of the histopathologist, but is also dependent on the selection of specimen from clinical material.

Although sensitiveness is high, reaching 95%, mistakes lead to false-negative results (Widmer 2001). The rest of the methods enable us to specify diagnosis and target antibiotic therapy better. Classic cultivation-taking is sufficient for objectification of the findings. We cannot expect any result during the surgery and its function lies in possible postoperative correction of the treatment.

A similar method, when the result is available after at least several hours, is – as mentioned above – the detection of bacterial RNA by real-time PCR procedure. A very controversial method seems to be microscopical assessment of bacteria on Gramm's colored sample; it has a number of false-negative results, because under the microscope we can detect bacteria randomly or only in massive and clinically entirely clear infection (Landor et al. 2005). Nevertheless perioperative cultivation is essential for identification of the agent. After clearing up the situation in the hip region we take at least three specimens from different spots and we send them for cultivation. By multiple withdrawal we improve the chance for positive cultivation and decrease eventual incorrect diagnosis of infection (Tsukayama et al. 1996).

Segawa recommends taking 5 perioperative samples for cultivation (Segawa 1999). Patel recommends 5 to 6 perioperative samples for cultivation. Each specimen taken we put through anaerobic cultivation, mycological examination and cultivation for TBC (Patel 2005). Ultrasound releasing of biofilm from arthroplasty is used for obtaining bacteria from the implant area (Tunney 1998). Sonification method is very well developed. Its major contribution is possible identification of sesil bacteria. Disadvantage of this method is complex with great demands on sterile transportation and sonification itself and therefore creates a major risk of contamination (Pilnáček and Bébrová 2002).

Single Antibiotic Therapy (Chronic Suppressive Therapy)

Treatment of infected arthroplasty by antibiotics only is not very effective. A major mistake is the administration of a broad range of antibiotics which are incorrectly used with great popularity as a first method of treatment. Deep infection of the joint replacement cannot be finally resolved by administration of antibiotics. It can lesson the symptoms but does not protect from bone loss, pain or limitation of the functions. It only covers symptomatology of acute inflammation, changes the infection into a chronic stage and postpones definitive solution with all negative consequences (Jahoda et al. 2000; Johnson et al. 1986; Spangehl et al. 1997; Vavřík et al. 2000). It is indicated only for patients unfit for surgical procedure and in patients who refuse operations even after repeated and thorough explanations.

Tsukuyama describes special indication for single antibiotic therapy when in the cases of surgical procedures of »presumable aseptic loosening« after reimplantation we get positive perioperative cultivation. In these cases we use appropriate antibiotics according to sensitivity for at least 6 weeks. This infection is very often caused by coagulase-negative staphylococci. Success rate of this therapy is 90% (Tsukuyama et al. 2003).

This procedure is sometimes called »chronic suppressive therapy«, when in this term we think only of controlled inflammation by long-term administration of antibiotics without surgical intervention. According to literature and in our opinion this process is uneffective (Bernard et al. 2004).

Debridement and Rinse Lavage

Debridement and rinsing lavage of infected arthroplasty combined with long-term intravenous antibiotic therapy are often related to treatment of early infection in case of fully integrated implants (Calton et al. 1997; Crockarell et al. 1998; Jahoda et al. 2000; Johnson et al. 1986; Tsukayama et al. 1996; Vavřík et al. 2000; Waldman et al. 2000). An operation is necessary up to two weeks after symptoms occur (Crocarell et al. 1998). The success rate of this method is according to literature between 17,9 and 71% (Calton et al. 1997; Crockarell et al. 1979; Jahoda et al. 2000; Johnson et al. 1986; Tsukayama et al. 1996; Vavřík et al. 2000; Waldman et al. 2000; Spangehl et al. 1997).

Fundamental break-throughs in this strategy have been worked out by Drancourt. In the treatment of early infection he uses revision and debridement together with a combination of rifampicine (900 mg/24 hours) and ofloxacin (600 mg/24 hours) after 6 to 9 months in cases of well-incorporated implants. The problem of loosened implants he solved by one-stage reimplantation and 5 months of administration of this antibiotic therapy. Indicated success rates, which are 81% at hip-joint replacement and 69% at knee-joint replacement, are surprisingly high. The effect of this treatment is attributed to high intracellular penetration of rifampicine and ofloxacin (Drancourt et al. 1993). An insignificant effect is a share of rifampicine on destruction of glycocalix and its influence in acidic environment (Cordero 1999).

In any case it is necessary to point out epidemiological risks related to long-term application of antibiotics. Especially rifampicine and fluorochinolones belong to medicines which have the ability to cause resistance relatively easy even during therapy. Combination of antibiotics should limit these risks, but in cases of several months of therapy would not absolutely decrease.

Our experiences are very similar (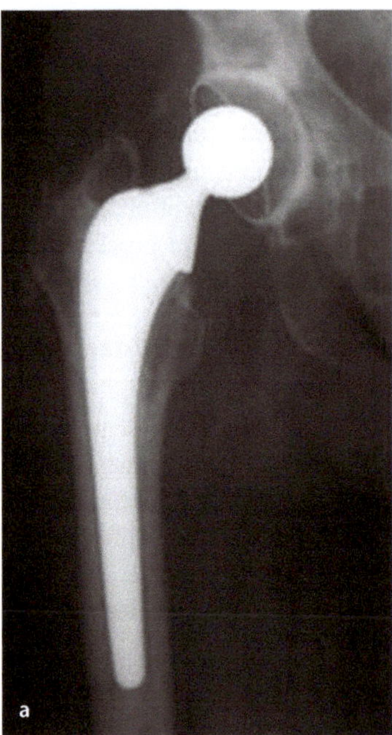 Fig. 7.3a,b). It is necessary to continue enthusiasm and not to indicate this procedure after expiration of time limits for indication of this method or even the use of antibiotic therapy only.

The success of this therapy depends on the time duration of infection is obvious. Debridement with retaining of implant in situ can be effective only with indication of surgical treatment until two, maximum three weeks from onset of symptoms and good function of implant. After this period it is necessary to choose a method with implant removal (Jackson and Schmalzried 2000).

A rather rare view is advanced from Trebse who recommends the use of revision, debridement and standard antibiotic therapy in stable implants in which infection does not last longer than one year, have no fistula, and well sensitive pathogen is known. Efficacy of this procedure when stability of the implant is examined at revision, debridement, lavage and suction drainage are performed, reaches 96% (Trebse et al. 2005).

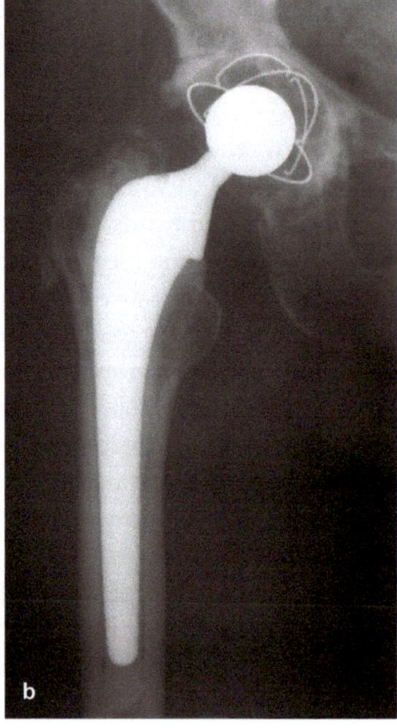

Fig. 7.3a,b. Radiologic documentation of successful one-stage reimplantation of hip-joint replacement performed for mitigated infection

One-Stage Exchange

Principle of one-stage exchange lies in the extraction of arthroplasty, careful debridement and reimplantation of new arthroplasty at one single operation (Bucholtz and Engelbrecht 1970; Calton et al. 1997; Jahoda et al. 2003; Raut et al. 1995; Spangehl et al. 1997; Vavřík et al. 2000). Long-term synchronous administration of antibiotics by sensitivity is a matter of fact. Successfully performed one-stage exchange reduces patient's treatment and costs (Buechel et al. 2004). One major problem of one-time procedure is that there is a sterile environment at the time of implantation of a new implant (Kraay et al. 2005). The advantage of one-time procedure is only one operation, shortening of hospital stay and lower internal risks, because of a much quicker return of function to the hip joint, and much lower therapy costs (Jackson et al. 2000).

This method was very popular in Europe in the past and the outcomes vary from 38,5% to 91,2% (Bucholtz et al. 1970; Calton et al. 1997; Jahoda et al. 2003; Raut et al. 1995; Spangehl et al. 1997; Vavřík et al. 2000). This trend is mainly shown in the U.S. where it is being left off for its poor score, when success rates reaches 70%. The cause of re-infection is seen in incomplete sterilization of bone bed (Gee et al. 2003). Wroblewski sets the effect rate of one-stage re-implantation up to 91% using bone cement with antibiotics. His protocol includes removal of infected implant, all bone cement, synovial tissue and capsule, repeated application of Betadine and re-implantation of a new implant by cement Palacos 40 g with gentamicin 0,5 g (Wroblewski 1986). Callaghan shows a one-stage re-implantation success rate of 91,7% at 10-year follow-up. A one-stage procedure is recommended in patients where pathogen is well known, has low virulence and good sensitivity for antibiotics (Callaghan et al. 1999). Lieberman reports about 91% success rate in two-stage procedure using cement with antibiotics (Lieberman et al. 1994). Raut informs about 84% efficiency in a study of 183 patients with hip-joint replacement infection treated by one-stage re-implantation (Raut et a. 1995). Ure shows a success rate of 100% in one-stage re-implantations of the infection of hip-joint replacement in a group of 20 patients. He uses cement with antibiotics. He emphasizes lower patients' stress and less costs than in two-stage procedure (Ure et al. 1998).

Within the last few years the one-stage procedure has become popular again. Jackson reviews 83% success in the files of his patients treated by one-stage exchange with the use of bone cement with antibiotics (Jackson et al. 2000). One-stage exchange is successful according to Bernard by 80% (Bernard et al. 2004). Wodtke presents 87,5% effectivity of one-stage exchange using non-cemented implants (Wodtke et al. 2005). Kraay reports of one-stage exchange results between 80 and 85% (Kraay et al. 2005).

Ideal candidates for one-stage exchange are patients with infection of arthroplasty caused by low-virulent organisms, glycocalix non-forming coagulase-negative staphylococci or non-betahemolytic streptococci (Marculescu et al. 2005). One-stage exchange is not recommended in running fistulas (Salvati et al. 1982). Although Raut does not agree with this opinion, he reports a 86% success rate in hip-joint replacement with running fistula.

From the above mentioned it is apparent that one-stage exchange has excellent outcomes in treatment of deep infection of arthroplasty only in certain cases. Schmalzried has set generally accepted selection criteria for indication of one-stage exchange (Schmalzried 1999): healthy patients with favourable status of soft tissues, preoperatively identified Gram-positive pathogen sensitive to antibiotics, minimum bone defect. These conditions of successful one-stage exchange were further developed by Jackson et al. (2000): absence of wound-healing complications of primary implantation, good health status of the patient, methicillin-sensitive coagulase-negative staphylococci, *Staphylococcus aureus* or *Streptococcus species*, pathogen sensitive to antibiotics possible to mix with bone cement. As a contraindication of one-stage exchange he states: polymicrobial infection, Gram-negative bacteria infection, especially *Pseudomonas species*, confirmed infection of methicillin-resistant strains of staphylococci and enterococcal infection.

A different point of view regarding one-stage exchange between Europe and the USA, is shown in recommendations by other American authors, which completely contrasts criteria, with previously mentioned selection above. Duncan suggests one-stage exchange in elderly patients, with poor health status, whose capability for two-time procedure is low (Duncan and Condon 2003). Nelson similarly recommends one-stage exchange for old patients and those who would not be physically able to undergo a two-stage exchange (Nelson et al. 2001). In our view this is a misleading opinion.

Important fact in using one-stage exchange is the necessity of precise performance. After extraction of infected arthroplasty and careful and large debridement it is necessary to put the antiseptic towel in the wound and close the wound temporarily. After rewashing in the operation theatre and retoweling the patient we can then perform exchange with new instrumentation. Non-cemented implants are not contraindicated because we can add proper local antibiotic carriers. It is essential to guarantee perfect primary fixation of the implant.

Two-Stage Exchange

Two-stage exchange is the most used procedure in treatment of deep infection (Booth and Lotke 1989; Calton et al. 1997; Duncan and Masri 1994; Garvin et al. 1999; Jahoda et al. 2000; Sculco 1992; Spangehl et al. 1997; Tsukayama et al. 1996; Vavřík et al. 2000; Whiteside 1994; Wilson 1990; Winsdor 1990; Younger et al. 1997). The success rate in hip-joint region is high. Garvin reviews a 95% success rate in a group of 40 patients cured by two-stage exchange, although he reports relatively high percentage of complications. Good results are reviewed by many others and their success rate varies between 90 and 96% (Booth and Lotke 1989; Calton et al. 1997; Duncan and Masri 1994; Garvin et al. 1999; Insall et al. 1983; Jahoda et al. 2000; Johnson et al. 1986; Sculco 1992; Spangehl et al. 1997; Tsukayama et al. 1996; Vavřík et al. 2000; Whiteside 1994; Wilson et al. 1990; Winsdor et al. 1990; Younger et al. 1997). Siebel shows 100% success rate of treatment of infected arthroplasty of the hip joint using spacer from bone cement with antibiotics (Siebel et al. 2002).

With the use of a new strategy the two-stage exchange remains the solution for real serious infections of the joint replacement. First steps are to considerate the extraction of arthroplasty, careful debridement, installation of rinsing lavage and long-term administration of antibiotics by sensitivity. The second step is the reimplantation after a period of time necessary for healing of infection. Best results are at two-stage procedure with a period of at least 6 weeks (Haddad et al. 2000).

For bypassing the period of time for eradication of infection the resection arthroplasty is used. Extremity is secured by external fixation or traction. This method markedly limits mobility of the patient, muscle atrophy and stiffness of other articulations develops. Damaged tissue fills up the space after extracted implant and in 80 to 100% soft-tissue contractures develop. Reimplantation is then very difficult because scars and contractures deform normal anatomy and the length difference of the extremity progresses very easily (Gee et al. 2003).

The application of a spacer is an improving contribution (◘ Fig. 7.4). Its major role is prevention from excessive contracture of soft tissues. It serves as support for the extremity and if properly formed in construction, the loss of the bone does not develop – on the contrary, bone quality improves (Booth and Lotke 1989; Calton et al. 1997). Well-formed spacers enable satisfactory mobility of the patient. If we use a spacer applied by intramedullary stem into medullary canal of the proximal femur, the spacer serves as armouring and protects femoral bone from fracture (Deshmukh et al. 1998). Using the ATB-impregnated cement, the spacer serves as a system releasing local antibiotics. For creating the spacer it uses cement with antibiotics, in our case Palacos with gentamicin, recently Copal. It is possible to use standard cement and mix in the antibiotic by sensitivity.

Kraay emphasizes the necessity of using an aggressive therapy, above all debridement. He does not hesitate to perform repeated revisions in cases of new infectious symptoms and remove necrotic tissues, heavy contamination or bone cement debris (Kraay et al. 2005). For us this is correct, but we assume that it is advantageous to use rinsing lavage, which removes well problematic minor debris from the articulation.

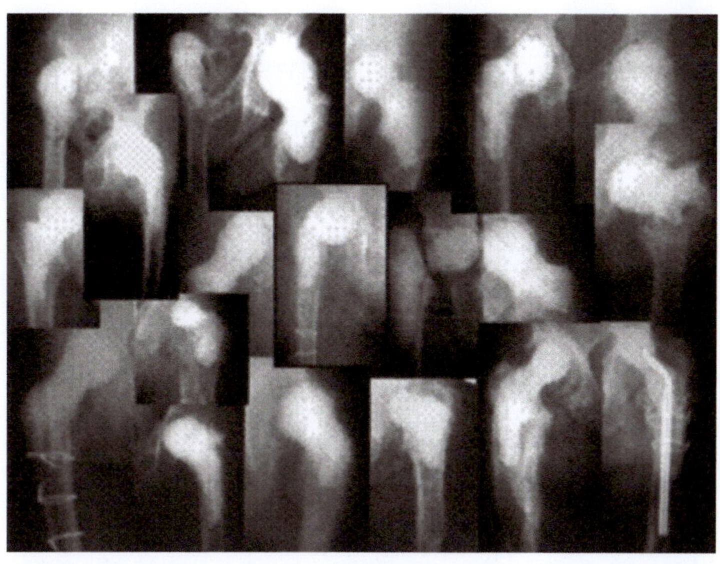

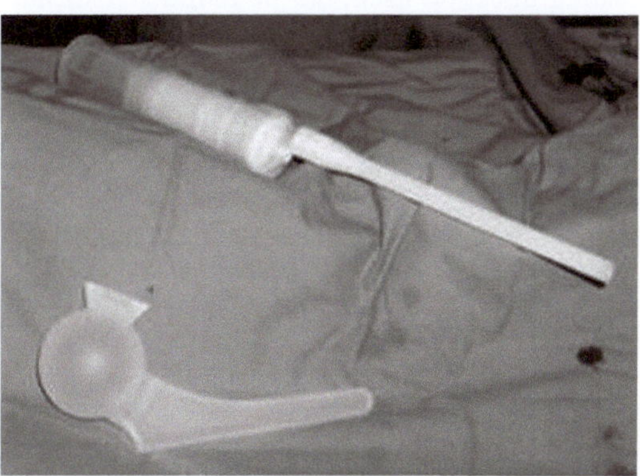

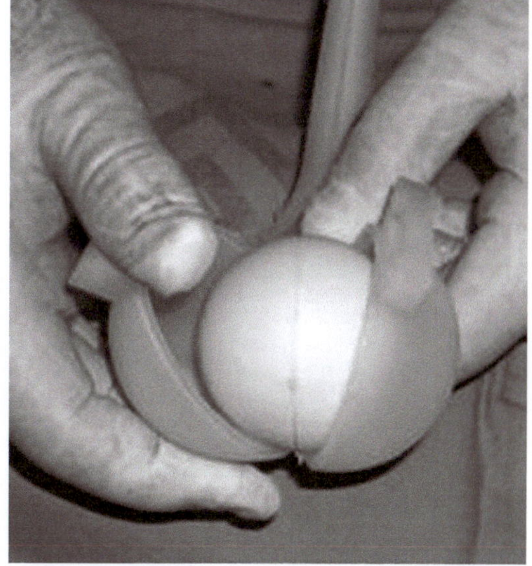

Fig. 7.4. Various shapes of manually formed spacers, used in the hip-joint region. It is apparent how shapes differ in relation to the technique of the surgeon

Fig. 7.5. Silicone shape for preparation of the hip spacer with cartouche filled up by bone cement with antibiotic

Fig. 7.6. Spacer is easily removable from the shape after setting

Classic rigid spacers are criticized for non-standard shapes, when its form depends on the skill of the surgeon and his craftsmanship.

For improving the qualities of shaped spacers many of us use various forms. There are now available systems of forms from silicone and some of them with armouring which enable certain standardization of the process. Silicone form for the hip joint usually has cervicocapital endoprosthesis shape and is available in various sizes. Form is filled up with vacuum-mixed bone cement with antibiotics from cartouche (Fig. 7.5). This process is relatively time-consuming but it brings satisfactory results (Fig. 7.6). The head of the spacer is thoroughly formed and smooth (Fig. 7.7). The risk of the fracture of the spacer remains at systems not using armouring.

Another possibility are so-called articulation spacers e.g. PROSTALAC. From 1989 on, Duncan began to use articulation spacers in the hip region with the first thought, to limit disadvantages of long stay of the patient on skeletal traction but also remove disadvantages of the classic spacers. At construction of the spacer he uses very thin poplypropylene sockets covered by a layer of cement with antibiotic, which is applied into acetabulum. The femoral component is made by templates where the body is made of stainless steel thoroughly wrapped in cement with antibiotic (Fig. 7.8).

After hardening of the spacer it is applied into the femoral canal as a press-fit implant. It is necessary to avoid integration of bone and cement. Duncan reports a success rate of 93,5% in a group of 86 patients at a two-year follow-up (Duncan and Masri 1994). Using the PROSTALAC method in the hip region, Younger reports a success rate of 94% in a group of 48 patients followed up for 43 months. Harris' hip score after operation was higher than 80 points in 80% of patients and increased by at least 30 points (Younger et al. 1997). Wentworth has experiences with the PROSTALAC system in 135 patients. Comparing literature, there are no statistically significantly better results from the point of view of healing infection itself, but he found statistically significantly higher rates of patients (97,3% vs. 88.1%, $p = 0,02$) with long-term functioning of the reimplanted arthroplasty. He assumes major advantages in restoration of hip-joint positioning, continuation or return of patient's mobility and less complex operation technique of reimplantation (Wentworth 2002).

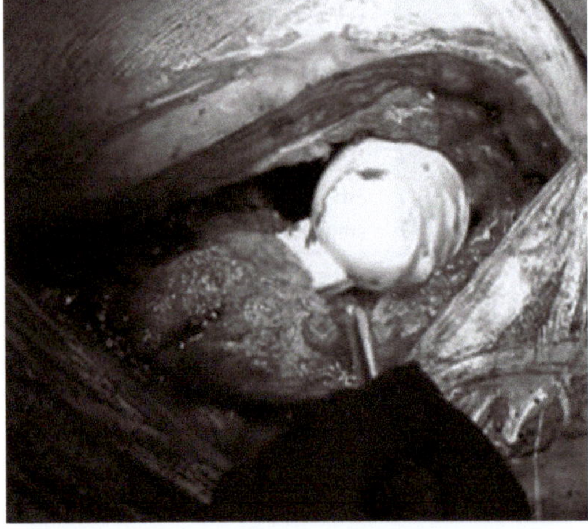

Fig. 7.7. Spacer can be applied or extracted easily

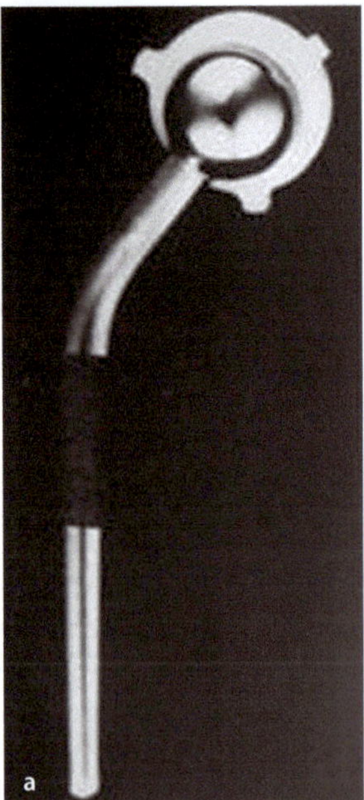

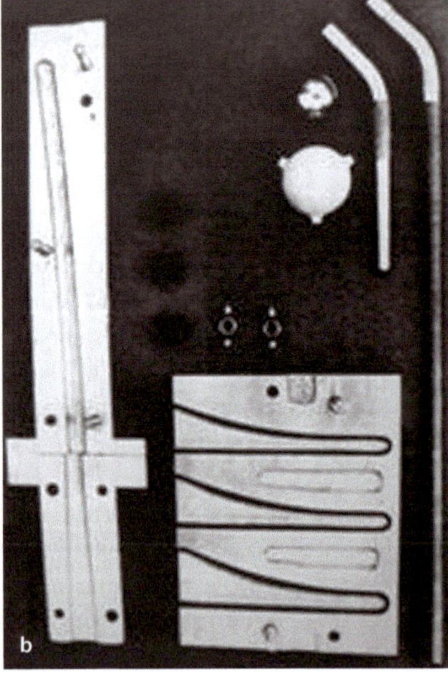

Fig. 7.8. a PROSTALAC implant.
b Complex instrumentation
PROSTALAC for cementless fixation

Regarding good results, it is very popular to use articulation spacers in some of our workplaces (Fig. 7.9). As a spacer the used resterlized endoprosthesis wrapped in cement with antibiotic is applied and inserted into the bone bed.

Excellent literature results and standardization of process, quicker physiotherapy and pronounced advance of patient's comfort have persuaded us of the convenience of using articulation spacers. Therefore, we have prepared and verified our own special implant which is only a temporary articulation insert for the time, essentially necessary for infection healing (Fig. 7.10). For its construction we used experiences from the creation of classic spacers and principles of our cannulated spacer enabling rinsing drainage of the medullary canal of the femoral bone.

Between 2002 and 2004 there were 26 patients with deep hip-joint replacement infection treated with an articulation-cannulated spacer. Healing of infection has been successful thus far. Time-duration of channelized articulation spacer hold in situ was 12,8 weeks. Harris' hip score showed excellent results, after reimplantation it reached on average of 94,7 points (89 to 99 points). The contribution of this method is much more proved by a mean increase of Harris' hip score preoperatively which was 37,5 points (26 to 72 points). Frequency of spacer complications and HHS increase are the fundamental differences in comparison with other methods that we use. Results of the patients in several groups were compared by a program with t-test ($p < 0,005$). Positive results of cannulated spacer are high success rates of the treatment of deep hip-joint replacement infection, less complications of treatment than in classic spacer methods, distinct comfort for the patients, excellent functional results of the treatment, standardization of operation technique, simple solutions within high modularity, and proven process of femoral canal drainage. Certain negative aspects can be found in its inability to fit into the large acetabular defects, necessity of patient's cooperation, and that the modular system can cause a higher risk of disintegration of the stem. The main problem is the relatively complex and technically demanding implantation.

An interesting solution can be the use of factory-made, so-called »ready-made« spacers from

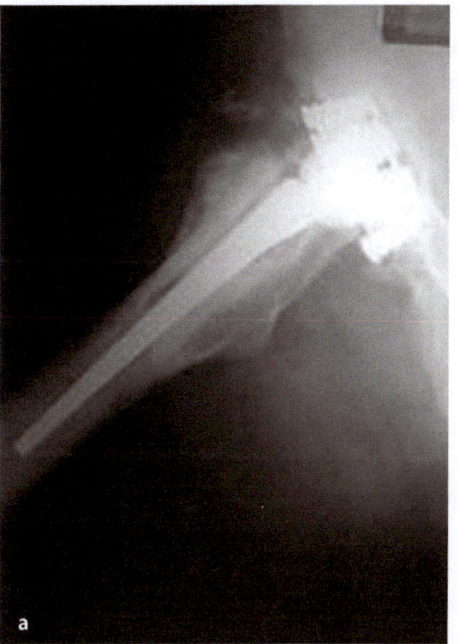
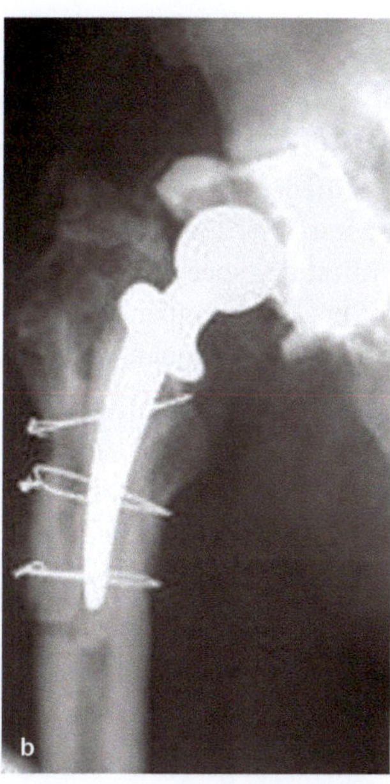
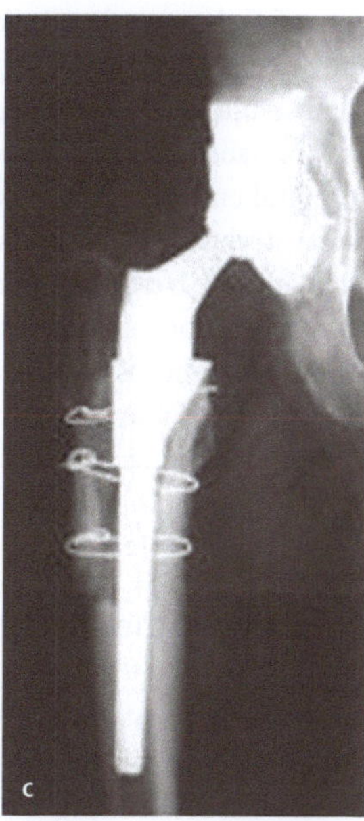

Fig. 7.9a–c. Using of articulation spacer in solving the infection of hip-joint replacement Balgrist/CF30 (Sulzer). Wagner approach was used for stem extraction. Articulation spacer is constructed using the small component Poldi. After infection recovery the socket Oblong was implanted, S-ROM stem (De-Puy)

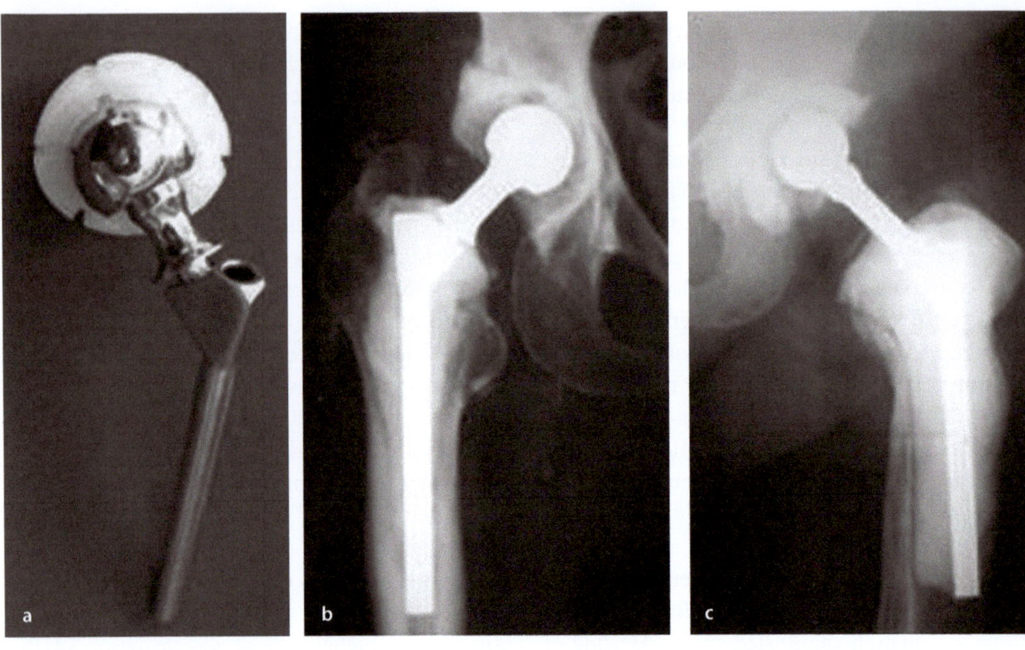

Fig. 7.10. a Cannulated articulation spacer – complete implant (at cooperation with ProSpon company), **b,c** X-ray of cannulated articulation spacer

bone cement with antibiotic. Preformed spacers, e.g. Spacer-K bring time reduction, standardization of technique, less mechanical complications and better functional results comparing with hand-made spacer (D'Angelo et al. 2005). Magnan uses prefabricated hip Spacer-G (Tecres) of cervicocapital endoprosthesis shape, stiffened by cylindrical steel nail. The success rate was 80%. The advantages are treatment standardization, speeding up of operation, and decrease of luxation number. Well-formed heads prevent for bone loss (Magnan et al. 2001). These prefabricated spacers are interestingly a technical solution. But its high price has limited, wider use of them for the moment.

Resection Arthroplasty

Resection arthoplasty is the actual extraction of the implant completed by thorough debridement of soft tissues, rinsing lavage and arrangements for preserving the stability of the extremity (Bittar and Petty 1982; Bourne et al. 1996; Cordero 1999; Duncan and Masri 1994; Kubiče and Pilnáček

1992; Spangehl et al. 1997; Vavřík et al. 2000). The keystone of resection arthroplasty is the creation of massive scar tissue necessary for painless motion and preserving of partial stability, which is reached by a long-term immobilization of the joint and by the application of skeletal traction (Fig. 7.11). It can be indicated as a first step towards two-stage exchange. As a final solution it is used in situations when there is no possibility for a procedure to be performed twice, for internal complications or no cooperation of those patients who are e.g. senile or have dementia or in technical inability for reimplantation for large bone-stock defects. It is suitable for patients who are not able to walk, patients with serious immune deficiency and drug addicts (Cordero 1999; Duncan and Masri 1994).

This procedure is well appreciated by only 40% patients on average (Bittar and Petty 1982). Subjective difficulties after resection arthroplasty of the hip joint are acceptable although the function is altered significantly. Pain of the hip joint after operation is reasonable, 80% of the patients state mild pain or medium pain which, however,

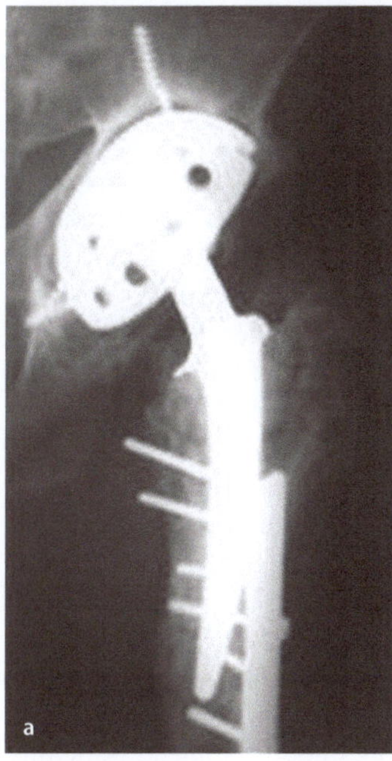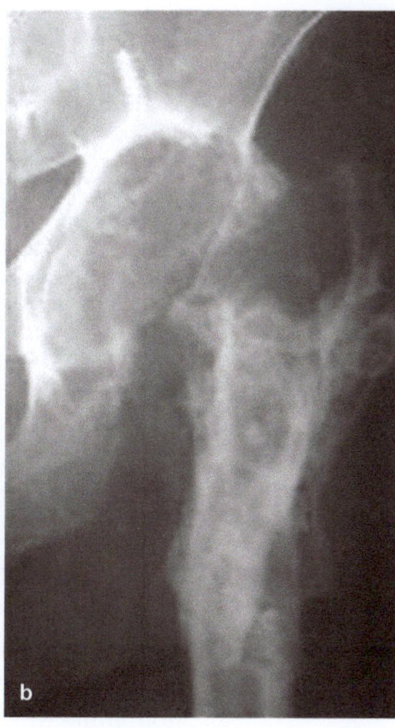

Fig. 7.11a,b. LOR/Poldi hip replacement with fistulating infection after reimplantation and osteosynthesis of periprosthetic fracture after trauma. Condition was treated by resection arthroplasty for internal complications

can be reduced by common analgetics, or complete painlessness (Hudec et al. 2005). Functional evaluation of the hip joint after resection arthroplasty is unfavourable. All patients suffer from claudications, and they cannot walk without support. In literature there are outcomes of resection arthroplasty from clearly bad to very good. An average of Harris' hip score oscillates between 63,2 points and 64 points (Hudec et al. 2005; Stoklas and Rozkydal 2004). The average shortening of the extremities in different authors varies between 3,7 to 6 cm (Hudec et al. 2005; Stoklas and Rozkydal 2004).

On the contrary we can find great differences in subjective evaluation of the patients from various authors. It ranges from 14% satisfied patients in the work of Petty et al. (1980) up to 100% satisfaction within the study of Böhler and Salzer (1991). Hudec states 78% of satisfied and partially satisfied patients, again comparable with the results of Bourne and Stoklas (Bourne et al. 1986; Hudec et al. 2005; Stoklas and Rozkydal 2004). Even an evaluation of hip pain after Girdlestone's procedure is considerably different as with various authors' results, 80% of painless cases with mild or medium pain of the articulation in the file of

Hudec is comparable with 84% of Stoklas and 79% of Štědrý (Hudec et al. 2005; Stoklas and Rozkydal 2004; Štědrý and Deniger 1987).

Conclusions

Prevention is the best strategy in the struggle with bacterial infection of joint replacements. Our responsibility for the patient does not end after the surgical procedure, but it is necessary to ensure prevention of late hematogenous infections. New technologies are being examined, e.g. the release of high doses of antibiotic »on demand« by new mechanism of ultrasound-initialized release. Other possibilities are the blockade of the communication of bacteria in biofilm, or the increase of sensitivity to antibiotics by destruction of biofilm by electrical field or ultrasound waves. Ehrlich describes futuristic conceptions of engineer approach to solution of biofilm questions by introducing so-called intelligent implants (Fig. 7.12). He suggests microelectromechanical systems (MEMS) which can be placed into joint replacements. Thanks to special sensors which detect RAP (ribonucleic

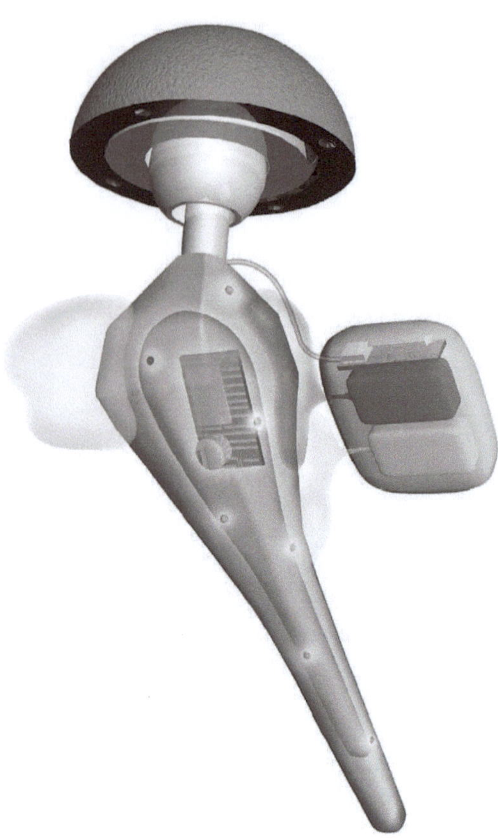

Fig. 7.12. Ehrlich recommends treatment by the smart implants which release a cocktail of pharmaceutical agents contained within integral reservoirs connected to the implant. Included in the reservoirs are pharmaceutical agents which give a molecular jamming signal that binds to the bacteria's receptors and contains a high dose of antibiotics (Ehrlich et al. 2005)

acid (RNA) III-activating protein) it is possible to identify bacterial infection and initiate treatment by means of telemetry after communication with your physician through bluetooth connection and internet. Ehrlich suggests a therapy by substances released from reservoirs in the implant, that interrupt the communication among bacteria on molecular basis and blind them. This prevents from toxin production and by repeated high doses of antibiotics eradicate planktonic forms of bacteria (Ehrlich 2005). Because these new, futuristic processes have been less effective so far or in the laboratory phase, there is no other way how to re-move the biofilm on the joint replacement than to remove the implant itself.

It is necessary to explain thoroughly to the patient all possible risks before the procedure. In case of infectious complications we can cooperate much better with well-informed but not scared patients. In the event of infection development the diagnosing must be as fast as possible.

There are many methods for the setting of the diagnosis. Individualization of the treatment helps us to gain the best possible results with the least demanding procedures.

Preoperative punction is very important for the verification of the diagnosis and for the selection of the best possible treatment method. To identify the pathogen we need prolonged cultivation and it is possible to use modern genetic methods like PCR. In cases of using only revision, debridement and lavage, we must keep indication limits which does not recommend using this method in other situations other than early infection stages, with an operation up to 2 to 3 weeks from onset of the symptoms. One-stage exchange is indicated only under strictly defined conditions. However, it shows very good functional results and is comfortable enough for the patient. It is useful to combine this procedure with qualities of a microbial agent, first of all according to its ability to create biofilm. Two-stage exchange is a solution for deep infections of the arthroplasty in remaining cases. The use of cemented spacer is an optimum way for preserving stability of the extremity during the period needed for infection healing, but also for holding enough space for future implantation of a new endoprosthesis. Spacers serve as a system for local antibiotic application by releasing from the bone cement and in the long term provides space for application of the rinsing lavage with antibiotic.

References

Barrack RL, Jennings RW, Wolfe MW, Bertot AJ (1997) The Coventry Award. The value of preoperative aspiration before total knee revision. Clin Orthop Relat Res 345: 8–16

Bernard L, Hoffmeyer P, Assal M, Vaudaux P, Schrenzel J, Lew D (2004) Trends in the treatment of orthopaedic prosthetic infections. J Antimicrob Chemother 53: 127–129

Bittar ES, Petty W (1982) Girdlestone arthroplasty for infected total hip arthroplasty. Clin Orthop 170: 83–87

Böhler M, Salzer M (1991) Girdlestone's modified resection arthroplasty. Orthopedics 14: 661–666

Booth RE, Lotke PA (1989) The results of spacer block technique in revision of total knee arthroplasty. Clin Orthop 248: 57–60

Bourne RB, Hunter GA, Rorabeck CH, Macnab JJ (1996) A six year follow-up infected total hip arthroplasty managed by Girdlestone's arthroplasty. J Bone Joint Surg 66-B: 340–343

Bucholtz HW, Engelbrecht H (1970) Über die Depotwirkung einiger Antibiotica bei Vermischung mit dem Kunsthartz Palacos. Chirurg 41: 510–515

Buechel FF, Femino FP, D'Alessio J (2004) Primary exchange revision arthroplasty for infected total knee replacement: a long-term study. Am J Orthop 33: 190 [discussion 198]

Callaghan JJ, Katz RP, Johnston RC (1999) One-stage revision surgery of the infected hip. A minimum 10-year follow up study. Clin Orthop 369: 139–143

Calton TF, Fehring TK, Griffin WL (1997) Bone loss associated with the use of spacer blocks in infected total knee arthroplasty. Clin Orthop 345: 148–154

Cordero J (1999) Infection of orthopaedic implants. European Instructional Course of Lectures 4: 165–173

Crockarell JR, Hanssen AD, Osmon DR, Morrey BF (1998) Treatment of infection with debridement and retention of the components following hip arthroplasty. J Bone Joint Surg 80: 1306–1313

D'Angelo F, Negri L, Zatti G, Grassi FA (2005) Two-stage revision surgery to treat an infected hip implant. A comparison between a custom-made spacer and a preformed one. Chir Organi Mov 90: 271–279

Deshmukh RG, Thervarajan K, Kok CS, Sivapathasundaram N, George SV (1998) An intramedullary cement spacer in total hip arthroplasty. J Arthropl 13: 197–199

Drancourt M, Stein A, Argenson JN, Zannier A, Curvale G, Raoult D (1993) Oral rifampicin plus ofloxacin for treatment of Staphylococcus – infected orthopaedic implants. Antimicrob Agents Chemother 37: 305–313

Duncan CP, Beauchamp C (1993) A temporary antibiotic-loaded joint replacement system for management of complex infections involving the hip. Orthop Clin North Am 24: 751–759

Duncan CP, Condon F (2003) Sepsis confirmed: what do you do now? Orthopedics 26: 931–932

Duncan CP, Masri BA (1994) The role of antibiotic-loaded cement in the treatment of an infection after a hip replacement. J Bone Joint Surg 76-A: 1742–1749

Ehrlich GD, Stoodley P, Kathju S, Zhao Y, McLeod BR, Balaban N, Hu FZ, Sotereanos NG, Costerton JW, Stewart PS, Post JC, Lin Q (2005) Engineering approaches for the detection and control of orthopaedic biofilm infections. Clin Orthop 437: 59–66

Garvin KL, Hinrichs SH, Urban JA (1999) Emerging antibiotic-resitant bacteria. Their treatment in total joint arthroplasty. Clin Orthop 369: 110–123

Gee R, Munk PL, Keogh C, Nicolaou S, Masri B, Marchinkow LO, Ellis J, Chan LP (2003) Radiography of the PROSTALAC (prosthesis with antibiotic-loaded acrylic cement) orthopedic implant. AJR Am J Roentgenol 180: 1701–1706

Goldenberg DL (1989) Infectious arthritis complicating rheumatoid arthritis and other chronic rheumatoid disorders. Arthritis Rheum 32: 496–502

Ha CW (2006) A technique for intraoperative construction of antibiotic spacers. Clin Orthop 445: 204–209

Haddad FS, Masri BA, Campbell D, McGraw RW, Beuchamp CP, Duncan CP (2000) The PROSTALAC functional spacer in two-stage revision for infected knee replacements. prosthesis of antibiotic-loaded acrylic cement. J Bone Joint Surg 82-B: 807–812

Hudec T, Jahoda D, Sosna A (2005) Středně- a dlouhodobé výsledky resekční artroplastiky kyčelního kloubu. Acta Chir Orthop Traumat čech 72: 287–292

Insall JN, Thompson FM, Brause BD (1983) Two-stage reimplantation for the salvage of infected total knee arthroplasty. J Bone Joint Surg 65(8): 1087–98

Jackson WO, Schmalzried TP (2000) Limited role of direct exchange arthroplasty in the treatment of infected total hip replacements. Clin Orthop 381: 101–105

Jahoda D, Sosna A, Landor I, Vavřík P, Pokorný D, Hudec T (2003) Dvoudobá reimplantace za užití spaceru – metoda volby při řešení infekce náhrady kyčelního kloubu. Srovnání metod užitých v letech 1979–1998. Acta Chir Orthop Traumat čech 70: 17–24

Jahoda D, Sosna A, Landor I, Vavřík P, Pokorný D (2004) Kanalizovaný artikulovaný spacer – funkční implantát pro řešení náhrady kyčelního kloubu. Acta Chir Orthop Traumat čech 71: 73–79

Jahoda D, Vavřík P, Landor I, Pokorný D (2000) Řešení infekce náhrady kolenního kloubu u pacientů s revmatoidní arthritidou. Čes Revmatol 8: 83–90

Johnson DP, Bannister GC (1986) The outcome of infected arthroplasty of the knee. J Bone Joint Surg 68-B: 289–291

Kraay MJ, Goldberg VM, Fitzgerald SJ, Salata MJ (2005) Cementless two-staged total hip arthroplasty for deep periprosthetic infection. Clin Orthop 441: 243–249

Kubiče J, Pilnáček J (1992) Odstranění infikované aloplastiky kyčelního kloubu. Acta Chir Orthop Traum čech 59: 294–296

Landor I, Vavřík P, Jahoda D (2005) Obecné principy léčby infekce kloubních náhrad. Acta Chir Orthop Traumat čech 72: 183–191

Lieberman JR, Callaway GH, Salvati EA, Pellicci PM, Brause BD (1994) Treatment of the infected total hip arthroplasty with a two-stage reimplantation protocol. Clin Orthop 301: 205–212

Magnan B, Regis D, Biscaglia R, Bartolozzi P (2001) Preformed acrylic bone cement spacer loaded with antibiotics: use of two-stage procedure in 10 patients because of infected hips after total replacement. Acta Orthop Scand 72: 591–594

Marculescu CE, Berbari EF, Hanssen AD, Steckelberg JM, Osmon DR (2005) Prosthetic joint infection diagnosed postoperatively by intraoperative culture. Clin Orthop Relat Res 439: 38–42

Nelson CL, Evans RP, Blaha JD, Calhoun J, Henry SL, Patzakis MJ (1993) A comparison of gentamicin-impregnated polymethylmethacrylate bead implantation to conventional parenteral antibiotic therapy in infected total hip and knee arthroplasty. Clin Orthop 295: 96–101

Parvizi J, Azzam K, Ghanem E, Valle CD, Barrack R (2008) Periprosthetic infection: A new prognostic classification. 27th Annual Meeting of the EBJIS. Barcelona, 2008

Patel R, Osmon DR, Hanssen AD (2005) The diagnosis of prosthetic joint infection: current techniques and emerging technologies. Clin Orthop 437: 55–58

Petty W, Goldsmith S (1980) Resection arthroplasty following infected total hip arthroplasty. J Bone Joint Surg 62(6): 889–96

Pilnáček J, Bébrová E (2002) Komplexní bakteriologické vyšetření při revizních operacích. 6. Národní Kongres ČSOT, Praha

Raut VV, Siney PD, Wroblewski BM (1995) One-stage revision of total hip arthroplasty for deep infection. Long-term follow-up. Clin Orthop 321: 202–207

Salvati EA, Chekofsky KM, Brause BD, Wilson PD Jr (1982) Reimplantation in infection: a 12-year experience. Clin Orthop Relat Res 170: 62–75

Santzen L, Carlsson AS (1989) The diagnostic value of C reactive protein in infected total hip arthroplasties. J. Bone Joint Surg 71-B: 638–641

Sculco TP (1992) Surgical treatment of rheumatoid arthritis. Mosby Year Book, St. Louis

Segawa H, Tsukayama DT, Kyle RF, Becker DA, Gustilo RB (1999) Infection after total knee arthroplasty. A retrospective study of the treatment of eighty-one infections. J Bone Joint Surg 81-A: 1434–1445

Siebel T, Kelm J, Porsch M, Regitz T, Neumann WH (2002) Two-stage exchange of infected knee arthroplasty with an prosthesis-like interim cement spacer. Acta Orthop Belg 68: 150–156

Schmalzried TP (1999) Careful patient selection is the key for direct exchange in the infected THA. Orthopaedics 22: 919

Spangehl MJ, Younger ASE, Masri BA, Duncan CP (1997) Diagnosis of infection following total hip arthroplasty. J Bone Joint Surg 79-A: 1578–1588

Stoklas J, Rozkydal Z (2004) Resekce hlavice a krčku kosti stehenní podle Girdlestona. Acta Chir Orthop Traum čech 71: 147–151

Štědrý V, Deniger J (1987) Funkce kyčelního kloubu po vyjmutí totální protézy. Acta Chir Orthop Traum čech 54: 141–145

Trebse R, Pisot V, Trampuz A (2005) Treatment of infected retained implants. J. Bone Joint Surg Br 87(2): 249–56

Tsukayama DT, Estrada R, Gustilo RD (1996) Infection after total hip arthroplasty. A study of the treatment of one hundred and six infections. J Bone Joint Surg 78-A: 512–523

Tsukayama DT, Goldberg VM, Kyle R (2003) Diagnosis and management of infection after total knee arthroplasty. J Bone Joint Surg 85-A (Suppl 1): 75–80

Tunney MM, Patrick S, Gorman SP, Nixon JR, Anderson N, Davis RI, Hanna D, Ramage G (1998) Improved detection of infection in hip replacements. J Bone Joint Surg 80-B: 568–572

Ure KJ, Amstutz HC, Nasser S, Schmalzried TP (1998) Direct-exchange arthroplasty for the treatment of infection after total hip replacement. An average ten-year follow-up. J Bone Joint Surg 80: 961–968

Vavřík P, Landor I, Jahoda D (2000) Zkušenosti s léčbou infektu aloplastiky kolenního kloubu. Acta Chir Orthop Traum čech 67: 121–127

Waldman BJ, Hostin E, Mont MA, Hunfergord DS (2000) Infected total knee arthroplasty treated by arthroscopic irrigation and debridement. J Arthropl 15: 430–436

Widmer AF (2001) New developments in diagnosis and treatment of infection in orthopedic implants. Clin Infect Dis 3 (Suppl 2): 94–106

Whiteside LA (1994) Treatment of infected total knee arthroplasty. Clin Orthop Relat Res (299): 169–72

Wilson MG, Kelley K, Thornhill TS (1990) Infection as a complication of total knee-replacement arthroplasty. Risk factors and treatment in sixty-seven cases. J Bone Joint Surg Am 72(6): 878–83

Windsor RE, Insall JN, Urs WK, Miller DV, Brause BD (1990) Two-stage reimplantation for the salvage of total knee arthroplasty complicated by infection. Further follow-up and refinement of indications. J Bone Joint Surg Am 72(2): 272–8

Wodtke J, Luck JFK, Loehr JF (2005) Failure analysis of 12 one-stage exchange procedures of THA for periprosthetic infection. Abstracts of 7th EFFORT Congress Lisbon

Wentworth SJ, Masri BA, Duncan CP, Southworth CB (2002) Hip prosthesis of antibiotic-loaded acrylic cement for the treatment of infections following total hip arthroplasty. J Bone Joint Surg 84-A (Suppl 2): 123–128

Wroblewski BM (1986) One-stage revision of infected cemented total hip arthroplasty. Clin Orthop 211:103–107

Younger AS, Duncan CP, Masri BA, McGraw RW (1997) The outcome of two-stage arthroplasty using a custom-made interval spacer to treat the infected hip. J Arthropl 12: 615–623

Zimmerli W, Trampuz A, Ochsner PE (2004) Prosthetic-joint infections. N Engl J Med 351: 1645–1654

Infection after Total Knee Artroplasty: Diagnosis, Management Strategies and Outcomes

Peter C.M. Verdonk, Pieter Vansintjan, René Verdonk

Introduction

Infection after Total Knee Arthroplasty (TKA) is the most devastating and challenging complication for both the surgeon and the patient to face. Although surgical techniques and treatment options have improved over the years, the overall risk for deep infection after TKA still remains 1–2% (Windsor et al. 1990; Bengtson et al. 1986; Bengtson and Knutson 1991; Gill and Mills 1991; Rand and Fitzgerald 1989). In case of infection, it is of great importance to quickly identify the problem and treat it adequately to minimize the risk of complications. A straight-forward management algorithm is the only way of dealing with infected implants properly.

Diagnosis of Infection

The diagnosis of an infected TKA is generally based on joint aspirates and cultures, laboratory results [Erythrocyte sedimentation rate (ESR), C-reactive protein (CRP)], radiography and clinical examination (Fehring et al. 2000; Emerson et al. 2002; Freeman et al. 2008; Calton et al. 1997; Wilde and Ruth 1988; Meek et al. 2004; Insall et al. 1983).

Classification of Infection

A clear classification of infection after total knee arthroplasty is needed to differentiate between acute and chronic, superficial and deep infection. This is of great importance when choosing a treatment option.

Identifying Organisms

Most common infecting organisms are Staphylococcus aureus, Staphylococcus epidermidis and Streptococcus species (Emerson et al. 2002; Calton et al. 1997; Meek et al. 2004; Insall et al. 1983; Rosenberg et al. 1988; Booth and Lotke 1989; Haleem et al. 2004; Hofmann et al. 1995, 2005; Haddad et al. 2000; Cuckler 2005; Anderson et al. 2008).

The host's healing capacity is vital (Jones and Huo 2006). McPherson et al. described the University of Southern California Staging System for prosthetic joint infections (Table 8.2; McPherson et al. 1997).

Management Options

When presented with the severe complication of chronic infection after TKA, there are a number of options available. Chronic suppressive antibiotics, irrigation and debridement with retention of components, one-stage re-implantation, two-stage re-implantation (early and late), resection arthroplasty, arthrodesis, and amputation have all been used in the past decades.

Chronic suppressive antibiotics and irrigation with debridement and retention of infected components have not been proven to eradicate chronic infection adequately (Freeman et al. 1985; Grogan et al. 1986; Johnson and Bannister 1986; Walker and Schurman 1984; Teeny et al. 1990; Marsch and Cotler 1981). It is also commonly accepted to use arthrodesis and amputation only as a last resort in treating infected TKA.

Different single- or two-stage methods have been developed in the past 3 decades, ranging from resection arthroplasty to a two-stage re-implantation with the use of an articulating spacer (Fehring et al. 2000; Emerson et al. 2002; Freeman et al. 2007; Calton et al. 1997; Wilde and Ruth 1988; Meek et al. 2004; Booth and Lotke 1989; Haleem et al. 2004; Hofmann et al. 1995, 2005; Haddad et al. 2000; Cuckler 2005; Anderson et al. 2008; Jones and Huo 2006; Johnson and Bannister 1986; Teeny et al. 1990; Falahee et al. 1987; Woods et al. 1983; Borden and Gearen 1987; Freeman et al. 1985; Burger et al. 1991; Goldberg et al. 1988; Beuchel et al. 2004). All of those techniques have shown good to excellent results in case series of patients presenting with infected implants.

Throughout the years two-stage re-implantation has been proven to be the most successful method of treating deep infection after TKA and is now the accepted gold standard of treatment. Once the diagnosis of infection is made, the first step consists of the removal of the infected implants, thorough debridement and copious irrigation. At that time there are 3 possible options:

1. irrigation and debridement without placement of any spacer;
2. placement of an AB-impregnated cementspacer block;
3. placement of an AB-loaded, articulating spacer.

Before reimplanting the new components, an interval is maintained during which the patient receives intravenous antibiotics according to the infecting organism. Different methods of rehabilitation are applied according to the first-stage procedure.

During the second stage a new total knee prosthesis is implanted using antibiotic-impregnated cement.

Both static spacer blocks and articulating spacers have been used during the interval in between the two stages. There is a growing trend towards the use of articulating spacers in favor of the static spacers. The former allow weight-bearing, provide functional range of motion during the antibiotic therapy and maintain the bone-stock quality whereas the latter have the risk of stiffening of the knee joint, compromising the bone stock and necessitating a more aggressive surgical exposure at second stage surgery.

In the following chapters, the results of different management protocols used for the treatment of infected total knee arthroplasty will be summarized. The questions that are still remaining will be debated in the discussion and finally an attempt will be made to draw a conclusion and make recommendations for clinical practice.

Materials and Methods

A search was performed using the MEDLINE database without language restriction, although only articles with abstracts in English were retained. Review articles, randomized controlled trials, retrospective cohort studies, case series, overview articles and case reports were systematically sought. We used the following search terms: »infection«, »infected«, »total knee arthroplasty«, »total knee prosthesis«, »management«, »spacer«, »dynamic«, »static«, »outcome«, »results«, »comparison«. There was no publication date limitation. Additional articles were identified from the reference list of retrieved reports and review articles.

Results/Clinical Studies

Diagnosis of Infection

As described earlier, there are different parameters that can be used for diagnosing infection after TKA.

The diagnosis of infection depends on the clinical appearance of the patient in the first place. The knee joint can present inflamed, red, swollen, tender on palpation, feeling warm and the patient can show clinical signs of systemic infection like fever, shivering, night-sweating, etc. Sometimes the only complaint patients have is continuous pain. This should be considered as an infection until proven otherwise.

Next to clinical presentation, all authors performed an aspiration of the possibly infected joint and put it into culture. One author advised that an aspirate with a white blood cell- count higher than 2500 with greater than 60% PMN is suggestive for infection (Mason et al. 2003). Most of the aspirations were performed preoperatively, some cultures were taken intraoperatively (Emerson et al. 2002; Freeman et al. 2007; Calton et al. 1997; Wilde and Ruth 1988; Meek et al. 2004; Rosenberg et al. 1988; Hofmann et al. 1995; Anderson et al. 2008).

When cultures remained negative, knees were presumed infected on the basis of cloudy or purulent joint fluid and/or when the pathologic evaluation showed acute inflammation (Emerson et al. 2002; Haleem et al. 2004; Hofmann et al. 1995, 2005).

Laboratory parameters mostly used to identify infection are erythrocyte sedimentation rate (ESR), C-reactive protein (CRP) (Emerson et al. 2002; Freeman et al. 2007; Calton et al. 1997; Meek et al. 2004; Hofmann et al. 1995, 2005) and sometimes a complete blood count (CBC) (Calton et al. 1997; Hofmann et al. 1995, 2005).

Radiography can also be helpful in diagnosing infection (Freeman et al. 2007; Wilde and Ruth 1988; Haleem et al. 2004; Hofmann et al. 1995, 2005). No one used routine nuclear scans.

Classification of Infection

Tsukayama et al. (2003) presented a classification of infection based on clinical presentation. (■ Table 8.1). They differentiate between *early, acute onset* (< 4 weeks post surgery), subdivided in superficial and deep, and *late, chronic onset* (> 4 weeks post surgery). The two remaining categories are: acute hematogenous infection and infection based on positive intraoperative culture. They use different management protocols, according to the classification of infection. For the specifics of their treatment we refer to the article. In none of the other articles included in the reference list, a specific classification for infection has been reported.

Infecting Organisms (and Host Factors)

The most common infecting organisms are Staphylococcus aureus and Staphylococcus epidermidis, followed by Streptococcus species (Emerson et al. 2002; Calton et al. 1997; Meek et al. 2004; Insall et al. 1983; Rosenberg et al. 1988; Booth and Lotke 1989; Haleem et al. 2004; Hofmann et al. 1995, 2005; Haddad et al. 2000; Cuckler 2005; Anderson et al. 2008). Other organisms were Escherichia

■ **Table 8.1.** Classification of infection based on clinical presentation

Classification	Diagnosis
I. Early postoperative infection	<4 weeks
A) Superficial	no extension through capsule
B) Deep	extension through capsule
II. Late chronic infection	> 4 weeks
III. Acute hematogenous	> 4 weeks
IV. Positive intraoperative culture	> 1 culture positive with same organism

Adapted and modified from Tsukayama et al. (2003).

Table 8.2. University of Southern California Staging System* for prosthetic joint infection

	Rating	Description
Criteria		
Infection type	I	Early postoperative infection (< 4 weeks postop)
	II	Acute hematogenous infection
	III	Late chronic infection (> 4 weeks postop)
Systemic immune status	A	Normal, uncompromised
	B	Compromised (< 2 compromising factors)
	C	Significant compromise (> 2 compromising factors)
		or one of the following:
		Absolute neutrophil count < 1000
		CD4 < 100
		Intravenous drug abuse
		Chronic infection other site
		Dysplasia/neoplasm of immune system
Local extremity status	1	Uncompromised (no compromising factors)
	2	Compromised (≤ 2 compromising factors)
	3	Significant compromise (> 2 compromising factors)
Compromising Factors		
Systemic		Systemic inflammatory disease
		Immunosuppressive drugs
		Infection/disease
		Renal and/or liver failure
		Diabetes
		Cardiopulmonary compromise
		Malnutrition
		Metastatic disease not of immune origin
		Chronic indwelling catheter
		Alcoholism or smoking
Local tissue		Reflex sympathtic dystrophy
		Multiple incisions or soft tissue loss from trauma
		Synovial cutaneous fistula (draining sinus)
		Subcutaneous abscess > 8 cm^2
		Vascular disease
		Prior fracture or trauma about joint
		Prior local radiation or infection > 3 months

* Clinical stage = infection type + systemic immune status + local extremity status. Adapted and modified from McPherson et al. (1997)

coli, Pseudomonas, Proprionobacterium acnes, coagulase-negative staphylococci, Acinetobacter species and others (Insall et al. 1983; Rosenberg et al. 1988; Booth and Lotke 1989; Hofmann et al. 1995, 2005; Anderson et al. 2008). In some cases multiple organisms were cultured (Rosenberg et al. 1988; Booth and Lotke 1989; Haleem et al. 2004; Hofmann et al. 1995, 2005; Anderson et al. 2008). Sometimes no organism could be cultured, antibiotics were then given empirically (Calton et al. 1997; Haddad et al. 2000; Hofmann et al. 1995, 2005; Anderson et al. 2008).

Management Options

Antibiotic Suppression +/– Debridement

Antibiotic suppression, either alone or in combination with surgical debridement and leaving the prosthetic components in place, is only adequate in the earliest and most benign infections (Freeman et al. 1985; Grogan et al. 1986; Johnson and Bannister 1986; Walker and Schurman 1984).

Teeny et al. (1990) treated 21 knees with irrigation and debridement leaving the infected components in place. Infection recurred in 15 knees. An increased infection rate occurred after irrigation and debridement in patients in whom the index prosthesis was in place more than 2 weeks. Subsequently they treated 9 knees with removal of the prosthesis, intravenous antibiotics and delayed re-implantation. There were no recurrences in this group (statistically significant). The authors concluded that irrigation and debridement is not likely to be successful for treatment of infections when used more than 2 weeks after the initial arthroplasty.

Treatment with AB alone has been reserved for the poorest of hosts and has had no success eradicating infection in another series (Marsch and Cotler 1981).

Debridement with retention of components has been a treatment with success in a high percentage of cases with acute infection with success ratings going from 11% to 83% (Grogan et al. 1986; Woods et al. 1983; Borden and Gearen 1987; Freeman et al. 1985). However, it has been shown in several series to be unsuccessful for chronic infections (Grogan et al. 1986; Borden and Gearen

1987; Burger et al. 1991; Hartmann et al. 1991; Schoicet and Morrey 1990).

Resection Arthroplasty

When resection arthroplasty is performed, the prosthesis and cement are completely removed with a minimal resection of bone and no attempt to obtain fusion. Postoperatively the knee is placed in a long cast or knee splint for several months. This procedure can achieve good infection control (Falahee et al. 1987), but functional results are undesirable and inferior to newer techniques. It can be a good alternative for arthrodesis (Cohen et al. 1988; Kaufer and Matthews 1986).

Single-Stage Treatment

Single-stage exchange arthroplasty has been successful in isolated cases of small series and has the advantage of less surgery, ability to maintain motion and soft tissue health and lower costs (Grogan et al. 1986; Teeny et al. 1990; Borden and Gearen 1987; Freeman et al. 1985; Buechel 1990; Göksan and Freeman 1992; Morrey et al. 1989).

Buechel et al. (2004) presented their series of 22 patients treated with primary exchange revision arthroplasties using AB-impregnated cement. The surgical technique consisted of excision of draining sinuses, complete synovectomy, removal of granulation tissue and debulking of the extensor mechanism. Postoperatively a cure of 4 to 6 weeks of parenteral AB and 6 to 12 months of oral AB was maintained. At an average FU of 10.2 years (range 1.4–18.6) 90.9% were free of recurrent infection. Knee scores averaged 79.5 with 85.7% good or excellent results. These results compare most favorably with those of delayed-exchange revision arthroplasty while providing a more cost-effective management program. The authors stressed that host condition was of great importance.

There have, on the other hand, never been shown good results in larger series (Johnson and Bannister 1986). Several studies have reported only up to 60% success in using this technique (Hirakawa et al. 1998).

Placement of AB beads or a block AB cement spacer gives the opportunity to deliver high dose local AB to the knee in concentrations higher than could be achieved with IV AB (Hofmann et al. 1995). This is why the single-stage treatment has been abandoned by most surgeons in favor of the two-stage treatment.

Two-Stage Treatment

There have been some reports of successful immediate re-implantation (Teeny et al. 1990; Borden and Gearen 1987; Freeman et al. 1985; Göksan and Freeman 1992) but the best results were obtained when this was delayed by at least six weeks with infection-control rates over 90% (Fehring et al. 2000; Emerson et al. 2002; Freeman et al. 2007; Calton et al. 1997; Wilde and Ruth 1988; Meek et al. 2004; Rosenberg et al. 1988; Haleem et al. 2004; Hofmann et al. 1995, 2005; Haddad et al. 2000; Cuckler 2005; Anderson et al. 2008; Jones and Huo 2006; Teeny et al. 1990; Borden and Gearen 1987).

The different sorts of late two-stage treatment can be roughly divided into three groups:
- irrigation and debridement without placement of any spacer;
- placement of an AB-impregnated cementspacer block;
- placement of an AB-loaded, articulating spacer.

Irrigation and Debridement without Spacer

Insall et al. (1983) presented the results of 11 two-stage re-implantations in a prospective study. They removed all components and cement and performed copious irrigation, then gave 6 weeks of parenteral AB and finally implanted a total condylar-type prosthesis. Large suction drains were left in the wound for 24–48 hours. Postoperatively a plaster in 5–10° of flexion was used and patients were allowed to walk with a walker, without weight-bearing (WB) four to seven days after the operation. The mean interval time was 52 days (range 38–82). At FU of 34 months (range 12–72), no patient had had a recurrence of the original infection, but 1 had a hematogenous spread from an infected bunion. The results were rated excellent in 5, good in 4 and fair in 2. Weakness of the extensor mechanism with an extension lag was the most frequent complication. They found that exposure for re-implantation could be difficult. Other complications were a DVT (deep vein thrombosis) in 3 patients and wound-healing problems in three others. The authors believe that AB alone is not adequate for the management of an infected prosthesis.

Rosenberg et al. (1988) treated 26 infected knees with debridement, prosthetic removal and 6 weeks of IV AB, followed by insertion of a new prosthesis. The average FU was 29 months (range 12–57). Al but four patients had os calcis skeletal traction for the first 3 weeks following debridement. Nine patients were treated without traction using simple immobilization. The initial group was treated with ROM exercises coupled with touch-down gait training. The latter group was allowed to ambulate in the bulky dressing 2–3 days after surgery, with ROM exercises 1–2 weeks after surgery. Re-implantation was performed between 6 and 8 weeks after removal. There was no evidence of residual infection at FU in any case. HSS at final FU showed 12 (50%) excellent results, 6 (25%) good, two (9%) fair and four (6% poor). Twenty-one knees had a ROM greater than 90° of flexion. Three had extensor lags of 20° and more. In 3 patients tibial tubercle osteotomy was required to prevent patellar tendon rupture. Two patients required flap coverage of an open wound. One patient developed a DVT. Keep in mind that the patients were always carefully chosen, so not everyone was suitable for their protocol.

A study by *Windsor et al.* (1990; continuation of the study by Insall et al.) with a two-stage protocol without using a spacer in between stages showed the results of 38 patients. The knee was immobilized for 6 weeks. They had an average FU of 4 years (range 2–10). There was only 1 documented recurrence of infection with the original organism, while 3 patients in whom the immunological system was suppressed had a subsequent hematogenous infection with a different organism. According to HSS, there were 11 excellent, 13 good, 6 fair and 7 poor results. Six patients needed a modified V-Y quadricepsplasty to obtain exposure. Osseous deficits frequently necessitated use of a custom-designed prosthesis with metal augmentation. Patellar bone stock was also often deficient. The results of the initial patients did not deteriorate with time. These results suggested that the 2-stage protocol for re-implantation with a six-week interval of IV AB is the procedure of choice for the treatment of an infection around a TKA. Some patients, however, had very complicated problems at the time of revision. It is important to note that, of the total of 48 patients that were seen because of infection, 27% were not candidates for this protocol.

In conclusion, it can be stated that early series without the use of an AB-impregnated spacer were encouraging, with reported success of 81–100%. However, re-implantations were difficult secondary to contracted soft tissues and poor bone stock and reported complications were significant (Windsor et al. 1990; Calton et al. 1997; Insall et al. 1983; Rosenberg et al. 1988; Borden and Gearen 1987).

Spacers

Many authors have reported their experience with either static spacers, dynamic spacers or both. In order to give an understandable overview of the results, a summary will be made of each step of the two-stage protocol, followed by the synopsis of the results obtained with the different sorts of spacers.

A. First-Stage

Wilde and Ruth (1988) reported their series of 15 patients treated with thorough debridement of infected tissue and components and placement of an AB-impregnated static cement spacer (polymethylmethacrylaat = PMMA) in 10 patients.

Since 1983 *Booth and Lotke* (1989) started treating infected implants with a two-stage exchange arthroplasty. The first stage consisted of debridement, implant removal and placement of an AB-impregnated polymethylmetacrylate (PMMA) spacer block. The cement was shaped like a tibial trial or like two flat bearing components to fill the knee extension gap. After copious irrigation the wound was closed in layers over suction drains.

Between 1987 and 1996 *Calton et al.* (1997) performed 25 two-stage re-implantations for sepsis. They performed a radical debridement of synovium, components and cement. Intraoperative radiographs were obtained to ensure complete cement removal. Rectangular cement spacer blocks were fashioned by hand to approximate the morphology of the tibia and maintain the knee in neutral alignment.

First-stage treatment in a series by *Haleem et al.* (2004) included removal of all prosthetic components and cement and placement of a static antibiotic-loaded cement spacer.

Hofmann et al. (1995) were the first to describe the use of an articulating spacer in between stages. During the 1st stage they performed a debridement, irrigation and removal of all components and cement. The articulating spacer was made by cleaning and autoclaving the removed femoral component during 10 minutes. This was reinserted during the same operation and articulated with a new tibial polyethylene (PE) insert. The autoclaved femoral component articulated with a new tibial polyethylen (PE) insert and in 40% of cases with a new all-PE patellar component of which the pegs were removed. The nonarticulating surface of the PE insert was coated with the AB cement mixture at a low viscosity state, which allowed the cement to adhere well. The cement was allowed to cure partially to a very doughy state and the remaining cement was applied. The component was then implanted, with care taken not to allow the cement to interdigitate into the bony surfaces by occasionally toggling the component until the cement was fully cured. This was repeated for the femur and the patella. The limb was taken to full extension in correct alignment and tension. The final curing allowed stabilization of the components to the bone. The wound was closed in layers without suction drainage to avoid leaching of AB.

Jones and Huo (2006) began using an articulating spacer as described by Hofmann et al. (1995) in patients with infected total joint arthroplasties in the mid 1980s. They also used antibiotic beads placed in the medial and lateral gutters and the suprapatellar pouch. No drains were used to allow high AB concentration levels in the knee and surrounding tissues.

Haddad et al. (2000) introduced their concept of articulated spacers in the late 1980s with the prosthesis of antibiotic-loaded acrylic cement (PROSTALAC). The spacer had femoral and tibial components, primarily made of AB-loaded Palacos bone cement with a small metal-on-polyethylene articular surface. Each prosthesis is made in the operating theatre using moulds before insertion. The design has evolved from a handmade facsimile to a sophisticated posterior-stabilised design. They also started with a thorough debridement of infected and necrotic tissue and removal of the prosthesis. Then femur and tibia were prepared in a similar manner to that for revision TKA. Once the cement had cured, the implants were removed from the moulds and cemented to the host bone, at a late stage of polymerization, to allow fixation without undue interdigitation of cement into the bone. When bone stock was good, press-fit fixation sufficed.

Meek et al. (2004) used the PROSTALAC articulating system during the first stage after radical debridement of all infected tissue.

Cuckler (2005) used the same protocol described by Hofmann et al. but also autoclaved the original PE in his series of 44 patients.

Anderson et al. (2008) conducted a retrospective study of 25 consecutive patients that underwent a two-stage articulating spacer surgery following the protocol described by Hofmann et al. A new PE patella was used in 12 cases (48%).

Fehring et al. (2000) compared a group of 25 patients with a static spacer with a group of 30 patients treated with a custom made AB-impregnated articulating spacer of polymehtylmethacrylate cement (PMMA-spacer). The latter was made using a stainless steel mold for the femoral component. A stemmed tibial baseplate was used in each patient. The tibial component was made flat to encourage ROM in the latest patients and had an impression with a femoral component trial made in the patients treated earlier.

Emerson et al. (2002) presented their results of 26 patients who received a static spacer block (SS) compared to 22 patients receiving a mobile spacer (MS). The traditional static acrylic cement spacer made of AB-impregnated Palacos was used in the first group, the MS was the same as described earlier by Hofmann et al.

Freeman et al. (2007) retrospectively reviewed medical records of all patients undergoing two-stage re-implantation for infection. Of 544 revision surgeries performed by the senior authors, 162 were due to infection and 133 were two-stage re-implantation procedures. 114 cases met their inclusion criteria. Static spacers were used in 38 procedures, while articulating spacers were used in 76 procedures. The first stage included aggressive debridement, removing all components and cement and performing a near complete syn-

ovectomy. Copious irrigation and implantation of an AB-impregnated cement spacer. Static spacers were fashioned as one solid block of AB-impregnated cement in extension. Articulating cement spacers were created according to the description of Fehring et al. (PMMA-spacer).

B. Antibiotics in Cement

Aminoglycosides were the antibiotic group most commonly mixed with the cement. Different concentrations were used ranging from 1.2 g to 3.6 g or 4.8 g per 40 g of (mostly Palacos) cement (Fehring et al. 2000; Calton et al. 1997; Booth and Lotke 1989; Hofmann et al. 1995, 2005; Haddad et al. 2000; Cuckler 2005; Anderson et al. 2008; Jones and Huo 2006). Vancomycin was sometimes associated to tobramycin in concentrations of 0.5–4 g per pack of 40 g cement (Emerson et al. 2002; Freeman et al. 2007; Haddad et al. 2000; Anderson et al. 2008; Jones and Huo 2006). One study reported the use of a combination of tobramycin, vancomycin and penicillin G in 1 patient (Haddad et al. 2000). In another study 3 patients had tailored antibiotics mixed with the cement according to the infective agent (Anderson et al. 2008).

C. Interval Period and (Parenteral) Antibiotic Therapy

Different authors almost all used different interval periods. There is one constancy and that is the use of intravenous antibiotherapy. Tailored antibiotics are usually given based on the cultured specimens and the resistance/sensitivity of the infecting organism, often in consultation with an infectious disease specialist or microbiologist (Fehring et al. 2000; Freeman et al. 2007; Calton et al. 1997; Wilde and Ruth 1988; Hofmann et al. 1995, 2005; Jones and Huo 2006).

Most studies agree on giving six weeks of tailored, parenteral antibiotics between the two stages with the patients being treated at home (Fehring et al. 2000; Emerson et al. 2002; Freeman et al. 2007; Calton et al. 1997; Meek et al. 2004; Booth and Lotke 1989; Haleem et al. 2004; Hofmann et al. 1995, 2005; Haddad et al. 2000; Cuckler 2005; Anderson et al. 2008; Jones and Huo 2006).

There were different parameters that were used to determine whether to proceed with re-implantation or not. Some authors used knee aspirations prior to re-implantation (Freeman et al. 2007; Wilde and Ruth 1988; Haddad et al. 2000), others relied on different combinations of laboratory results (CRP, ESR, CBC), clinical appearance, soft-tissue assessment and bone scan (Fehring et al. 2000; Emerson et al. 2002; Freeman et al. 2007; Booth and Lotke 1989; Cuckler 2005).

In some studies, re-implantation only was carried out after a drug-free holiday ranging from 2–6 weeks (Freeman et al. 2007; Hofmann et al. 1995, 2005; Haddad et al. 2000). In others, the antibiotics were continued chronically in some patients (Hofmann et al. 1995, 2005) or until the intraoperative cultures were negative (Fehring et al. 2000).

D. Rehabilitation Between Stages

Rehabilition protocols, although very important in revalidation, were not always reported. Two groups can be distinguished; the patients that were immobilized by cast or plaster shell after the first stage and the patients that were allowed range of motion (ROM) after first-stage surgery. Those two groups correspond with the static spacers and articulating spacers respectively.

Surprisingly, most patients in whom an articulating spacer was implanted also were immobilized for 5 to 10 days before ROM was allowed (Hofmann et al. 1995, 2005; Jones and Huo 2006) this to ensure adequate wound healing. In most studies, ROM exercises, CPM or physical therapy were not allowed until the wounds had properly healed (Fehring et al. 2000; Emerson et al. 2002; Freeman et al. 2007; Hofmann et al. 1995, 2005).

Another study in which articulating spacers were implanted encouraged the patients to actively mobilize immediately following surgery (Meek et al. 2004).

In one study patients were allowed to weight-bear and motion as tolerated. By the time of 8 weeks postoperatively, 95% were full WB without assisting devices (Cuckler 2005). In another recent study following the first stage, patients were encouraged to mobilize as much as could be tolerated. CPM (continous passive motion) was used and physical therapy ordered on the same day, immediately post procedure. Patients were maintained on partial WB with a walker or forearm crutches (Anderson et al. 2008).

Concerning weight-bearing (WB) protocols ranged from touchdown (Fehring et al. 2000) and partial WB (Anderson et al. 2008) to 50% WB with a walker or crutches (Freeman et al. 2007; Hofmann et al. 1995, 2005; Jones and Huo 2006) or even full WB as tolerated (Cuckler 2005). Weight-bearing decreases osteoporosis of disuse.

E. Second-Stage Reconstruction

After the interval period, the patients were examined and the decision was made whether to proceed with the second-stage re-implantation or not.

As described above, the time between first- and second-stage surgery varied a lot from study to study.

At second-stage surgery, the spacers were removed and a new total knee prosthesis was implanted. Antibiotic impregnated cement was routinely used.

F. Results

Early re-implantation within 2 weeks of joint removal and debridement have been 35% to 48% successful with eradication of infection (Morrey et al. 1989; Laskin 1976; Petty et al. 1975).

Static Spacers. Fifteen patients of which 10 received a static cement spacer (PMMA) were followed for more than one year by *Wilde and Ruth* (1988). The average age at re-implantation was 68 years (range 49–82); 8 men and 7 women were evaluated. HSS (Hospital for Special Surgery) Knee Score was 75.5 points (range 48–94); average flexion was 81° (range 52–120) and average extension was +6° (range 0–30). There were a number of serious complications: DVT in 4 patients, high probability of pulmonary embolism in 2 patients, superficial wound dehiscence in 3 patients and greater than 6 days of serous or hematoma drainage in 4 patients. The success rate in controlling infection was 80% overall and 90% when an AB spacer was used, although not statistically significant.

Booth and Lotke (1989) presented their results of 25 patients with an average age of 67 years (range 31–89) and FU of 25 months (range 6–59).

There were 13 women and 12 men. They had only 1 failure, giving a success ratio of 96%. Five patients had severe wound-healing problems. The subjective results were excellent in 21, good in 2 and fair in only 1 patient. HSS scores were average 81.5 and 64 for function (ranges 55–95 and –20 to 100). Knee motion was obviously less than primary TKA, but a surprising number of patients were left with functional knees and were delighted with the result. Flexion averaged 100° (range 20–120). Flexion contracture was more apparent than extension lag. Seven patients had a 0–5° extension loss, but the loss of motion was not proportional to the duration of the spacer block immobilization. In addition, the second-stage reconstruction exposure and procedure were difficult because of soft tissue contractures.

Calton et al. (1997) treated 25 knees in 24 patients with a static cement spacer block. The average interval time was 56 days. The average FU was 36 months (range 14–72); 13 patients were women, 11 were men. Sixteen knees had constrained condylar implants and nine had posterior stabilized implants. Wedges or blocks were used in 18 cases. There were two cases of reinfection giving an eradication of 89%. They specifically assessed the amount of bone loss and saw that tibial and femoral bone loss frequently occurred from invagination of the spacer block into the cancellous bone. Tibial bone loss was present in 10 (40%) of cases and averaged 6.2 mm, femoral bone loss occurred in 11 (44%) of cases and averaged 12.8 mm. Bone loss was more common when spacer blocks were undersized.

Haleem et al. (2004) reported the mid-term to long-term results of 96 knees in 94 patients treated with a 2-stage re-implantation and static spacer block between stages. There were 50 men and 44 women with a median age of 69 years (range, 37-89) at the time of re-implantation. Median FU was 7.2 years (range, 2.5-13.2). At latest FU 62 patients were still alive and 32 had died. Three patients died fewer than 2 years after their re-implantation and 1 was lost to FU. None of these had evidence of infection at latest FU. Fifteen knees (16%) required reoperation, 9 (9%) for reinfection, 6 (6%) for aseptic loosening. The estimated survivals free of reoperation for infection were 93.9%

and 85% at 5 and 10 years respectively. Of the 9 infected knees, 5 had an additional 2-stage protocol and all were infection free at final FU. Two had an above knee amputation and two had successful arthrodesis. The mean time between index arthroplasty and resection arthroplasty was 26.2 months (range 0,5-177). The preoperative KSS pain and function scores improved significantly. Pain scores from a median of 49 point (range 4-85) preop to a median of 89 points (range 35-97) postop. Preop function scores went from 5 (range 0-80) to 50 points (range 0-100) postop. The preop ROM had a median of 85° (range 30-125) and 90° (30-120) at latest FU. All of these improvements were statistically significant.

Articulating Spacers. In a series of 26 patients (14 M/12 F) with an average age of 70 years (range 40–80), *Hofmann et al.* (1995) saw that no patient had positive cultures at the time of re-implantation. One patient died of pneumonia 1 month after spacer placement. There had been *no recurrences* of infection with an average FU of 31 months (range 12–70). At secondstage, the articulating spacers could be easily removed by hand or by gentle tapping with a disimpactor. The soft tissues appeared supple and healthy and bone quality was good in all patients. Frozen tissue sections were used to decide to proceed with the re-implantation (< 5 PMN white cells per HPF). None showed acute inflammation, therefore, all were reimplanted. The modified HSS scores improved from 57 preoperatively to 88 postoperatively (average improvement of 31 points). Excellent results were seen in 72%, good in 20%, fair in 8%, no patients had poor result. The average ROM before re-implantation was 10–80°, while ROM at latest FU was 5–106° (average improvement of 30°). Pain scores averaged 35 (out of 40) at latest FU. No wound-healing problems, no difficulty with exposure at re-implantation and no DVT with pulmonary embolism were encountered.

They reported results of an extended series of 50 patients with an average age of 67 years (38–92). The average FU was 74 months (24–150). No patients were lost to FU. Eleven patients had died with an average FU of 48.5 months. The average interval time with spacer was 12 w (4–58). There were 6 (12%) recurrent infections at an average of 35 months (7–60) after re-implantation. Three out of those six had diabetes mellitus. All of those patients were treated with repeat articulating spacers. Two were doing well, one died 3 years later free of infection and the remaining two died from medical complications in the perioperative period after their second articulating spacer placement.

All the spacers were stable, but could again be easily removed by tapping with a mallet and punch. During second-stage operation, soft tissues were compliant in all 50 patients with minimal adhesions and excellent exposure. The tourniquet time was 77 minutes (range 42–119) for debridement and spacer placement, 73 min (range 33–120) for re-implantation. Again none of the patients had positive cultures at the time of re-implantation.

The modified HSS was 64 points (30–85) before debridement and improved to 89 points (70–100) after re-implantation. This was an average improvement of 25. Excellent results were seen in 70%, good in 20%, fair in 8%, 1 (2%) had a poor result and was converted to an arthrodesis (Hofmann et al. 2005).

Of 54 patients who underwent a two-stage revision using the PROSTALAC system by *Meek et al.* (2004), 7 had died by the time of FU, *none had infection*. They were compared with an aseptic revision group of 55 patients. The average FU was 41 months. There was no bone loss in the septic group. Two patients (3.7%) had recurrence of infection giving a success ratio of 96.3%. None of the postoperatively measured outcomes demonstrated the septic revisions to be statistically worse than the aseptic revisions.

Haddad et al. (2000) included 45 of 59 patients with infected knee arthroplasty in their series. One patient was too ill for second-stage procedure, 2 patients died and had no evidence of recurrent infection. No patient was lost to FU. There were 19 men and 26 women, with a mean FU of 48 months (range 20–112). The mean age was 69 years (26–83). Drainage or debridement had been undertaken elsewhere in 26 and 16 had discharging sinuses. Earlier versions of the PROSTALAC spacer were used in 22 patients, 23 patients received the new version. The mean interval was 15.5 weeks (3.3–96.7). Four patients had recur-

rence of infection, giving a 91% overall control of infection. Initially ESR and CRP levels were not measured, but now this is standard procedure. The main advantage of the approach, according to the authors, was the relief of pain between stages. The HSS score went from 42.4 on presentation to 55.9 at first stage and to 71.4 at final FU. These improvements were significant. The ROM seen in the interval period confirmed a maintained mobility. There was a small residual extensor lag at final review. Most complications were related to the extensor mechanism and occurred in the subgroup of patients treated with the old PROSTALAC spacer design. In 1 patient a latissimus-dorsi transfer was needed for wound problems.

Forty-four chronic infections with an average age of 68 years (44–92) were treated with an articulating spacer by *Cuckler* (2005). There were 31 women and 13 men with an average FU of 5.4 years. The average ROM was 110° (range 45–125) at 12 weeks after debridement. The average Knee Society Score before debridement was 36 (range 7–48); at 1 year after re-implantation it had improved to 84 (range 45–98). ROM at 1 year averaged 112° (range 45–125). There was no statistically significant difference between ROM after placement of the articulated spacer and ROM after revision. No patient required a quadriceps snip or other similar procedures to enhance exposure. Four patients were so comfortable that they delayed a second stage conversion more than 1 year. There has been only 1 failure in this series.

Jones and Huo's (2006) initial clinical experience with 23 patients was 22 (96%) free of infection after a mean FU of 13 months (range 3–27). One patient (type C) had recurrence of infection and was treated with amputation.

Anderson et al. (2008) included 25 consecutive patients with infected primary TKA in their retrospective study. Fifteen women and 10 men with a mean age of 64 years (range 45–87) with a mean FU of 54 months (range 24–108). One patient (4%) had recurrence of infection with the same organism, giving a success rate of 96%. He was finally treated with fusion and external fixation. The average ROM prior to re-implantation was 5–112° and at latest FU averaged 2–115°. Modified HSS before first stage were a mean of 60 points (range 27–80) Immediately before re-implantation the mean score was 68 (range 35–80) and at latest FU a mean of 91 (range 65–100) was observed. All but one patient received constraint prostheses. No difference in outcome was seen between patients who had a new patellar component between stages and those who did not. No complications of DVT or PE, or delayed wound healing were encountered in this series.

Articulating vs. Static Spacers. In a retrospective study by *Fehring et al.* (2000), 25 patients were treated with static nonarticulating spacers (SS) versus 30 patients treated with tobramycin-laden articulating spacers (AS)(PMMA spacer). One patient was lost to FU in each group. The average FU in the SS group was 36 months (range 24–72) versus 27 months in the AS group (24–36). Three patients in the SS group and 1 patient in the AS group died during the studie period. In the SS group, 3 (12%) TKA became reinfected versus 1 (7%) in the AS group giving an eradication rate of 86% and 92%, respectively. These differences were not statistically significant. Fifteen of 25 (60%) in the SS group had unexpected bone loss between stages. Each bone defect was an exact imprint of the spacer block. No bone loss could be measured in the AS group. Bone loss was correlated with the length of time of the interval period (48 days for patients without bone loss versus 88 days for patients with bone loss). HSS score was 83 points (37–98) and 84 points (45–95) in the SS and AS group respectively. ROM at final FU averaged 98° (SS, range 50–120) and 105° (AS, range 90–126). Both differences were not statistically significant, maybe due to low power ($\beta = 0.29$), but there was a medium effect size for ROM, indicating a possible clinically significant trend. The average operative time was 219 minutes (SD 48 min) in the SS group and 240 minutes (SD 45 min) for the AS group. Again there was no significant difference. There was also no difference between groups in the need for extensile exposure techniques. One snip and one V-Y plasty were used in the SS group, two snips were used in the AS group.

Emerson et al. (2002) compared 26 static with 22 mobile, articulating spacers (as described by Hofmann et al). The FU of the block spacers aver-

aged 7.5 years (range 2.8–12.7), those of the mobile spacers 3.8 years (2.6–6.4). Six patients died in the SS group, 1 patient died in the MS group. There was no significant difference in preoperative knee flexion (79.3° vs 73.4°, SS and MS). At final FU the SS achieved an average of 93.7° and the MS 107.8°, which was statistically significant. Reinfection rate was designated as acute within 3.6 years from the re-implantation and late after 3.6 years. It was not significantly different within the acute stage between both groups (7.6% vs 9%) giving success rates of 92.4% and 91%. Late reinfection could only be evaluated in the SS group. It was linear with time. The final rate was 30.7% (8/26) with all infections caused by new organisms. Bone loss was not specifically evaluated, but did not seem a problem with either type of spacer. There were no technical complications of either spacer techniques that compromised the second-stage reconstruction. Mobile spacer components required more time and care in the removal process compared with the acrylic block spacer. The knee tissues of the MS group were demonstrably more supple at re-implantation than in the SS group.

Freeman et al. (2007) retrospectively reviewed medical records of all patients undergoing two-stage re-implantation for infection. Of 544 revision surgeries performed by the senior authors, 162 were due to infection and 133 were two-stage re-implantation procedures. 114 cases met their inclusion criteria. Static spacers were used in 38 procedures, while articulating spacers were used in 76 procedures (PMMA spacer). Mean age of the patients was 68 years (range 38–91) with 50 men and 59 women. Of the 109, 35 were excluded because not enough data were available. The final dataset included 76 procedures in 74 patients with an average age of 67 (range 41–87). Static spacers (SS) were used in 28 procedures, articulating (AS) in 48. The average FU was 71.2 months (range 24–196); SS group had a FU of 86.6 months (range 24–196.3) and AS 62.2 months (25.7–119.6). There was a statistically significant difference in average age between the SS group with 71.2 years and the AS group with 64.9 years. The reoperation rate for infection was 5.3% in the AS group and 7.9% in the SS group (not significant) giving success ratios of 92% for SS and 95% for AS. There were no significant differences in KSS pain scores. The median KSS pain score was 45 versus 50 for the AS and SS group respectively. The postoperative KSS function scores were higher in the AS group; 70 versus 45, but not significantly different. When the 4 subcategories were analyzed separately, the articulating group had a significantly higher percentage of patients with good to excellent functional results than the static group. When interpreting these results, one should beware of the age difference, AS had younger patients, which could result in better functional scores.

Discussion

Over the years, many different techniques have proven their use in the treatment of an infected total knee arthroplasty.

Back in 1983 Insall et al. already knew the critical importance of antibiotic management. They suggested that an infectious disease consultant should be regularly consultated and be involved in the therapy. This advise has been followed by almost all authors, and many advise frequent consultation with either an infectious disease specialist or a microbiologist.

Evolving techniques have allowed us to treat patients with intravenous antibiotics at home, allowing a significant decrease in the length of hospitalization (Rosenberg et al. 1988).

Leaving the infected components of a total knee in place and treat them with antibiotic suppression, either alone or in combination with surgical debridement has only be proven adequate in the earliest and most benign infections (Freeman et al. 1985; Grogan et al. 1986; Johnson and Bannister 1986; Walker and Schurman 1984; Teeny et al. 1990).

Although Buechel et al. had great success with a single-stage primary exchange revision, it should be noted that not all patients were admitted for their treatment protocol. Single-stage exchange arthroplasty has been successful in isolated cases of small series and has the advantage of less surgery, ability to maintain motion and soft-tissue health and lower costs (Fehring et al. 2000; Emerson et al. 2002; Freeman et al. 1985; Johnson and Bannister 1986; Borden and Gearen 1987). There have, on the other hand, never been shown good results in larger series. Several studies have reported only up to 60% success in using this technique (Hirakawa et al. 1998).

Placement of AB beads or a spacer gives the opportunity to deliver high-dose local AB to the knee in concentrations higher than could be achieved with IV AB (Hofmann et al. 1995). This is why the single-stage treatment has been abandoned by most surgeons in favor of the two-stage treatment.

When one chooses for a second-stage approach, one has the option of placing no spacer, a static spacer or a dynamic spacer at first-stage surgery.

Early series without the use of an AB-impregnated spacer were encouraging, with reported success of 81–100%. However, re-implantations were difficult secondary to contracted soft tissues and poor bone stock, often necessitating custom-designed implants. Moreover, reported complications were significant (Rand et al. 1986; Rand and Fitzgerald 1989; Calton et al. 1997; Insall et al. 1983; Rosenberg et al. 1988; Borden and Gearen 1987).

Although Booth and Lotke (1989) found a surprisingly good bone quality after an interval period with a *static spacer*, loss of bone stock was not assessed. Other studies report good clinical and functional outcomes with static spacers, but high complication rates exist. Bone loss up to 40–60% of cases (Fehring et al. 2000; Calton et al. 1997), deep vein thrombosis and pulmonary embolism (Wilde and Ruth 1988), wound problems (Wilde and Ruth 1988), difficulty of exposure at second stage due to capsular contracture and significant scarring (Fehring et al. 2000) and spacer-block migration and invagination in the cancellous bone (Haleem et al. 2004) have all been reported. The use of a static spacer block between stages had become an accepted practice. But patients are inconvenienced with the inability to bend the knee or bear any significant weight during the interim period.

Treating infection after TKA with use of articulating spacers has also shown excellent eradication of infection, equal to static spacers, combined with improved range of motion and function. The mobile spacer as described by Hofmann et al. is the most commonly used (Emerson et al. 2002; Hofmann et al. 1995, 2005; Cuckler 2005; Anderson et al. 2008; Jones and Huo 2006).

Other spacers with equal eradication results are the PROSTALAC (Meek et al. 2004; Haddad et al. 2000) and PMMA spacers (Fehring et al. 2000; Freeman et al. 2007; Anderson et al. 2008).

Articulating spacers in general have the advantages that they allow motion and partial weight-bearing during the interval period, which promotes a healthy and supple soft-tissue sleeve. This improves wound healing, allows easier re-implantation, improves bone quality and ROM. The patient is left with a functioning knee before re-implantation that allows mobility and may diminish complications (Hofmann et al. 1995, 2005; Fehring et al. 2000; Emerson et al. 2002; Freeman et al. 2007; Cuckler 2005; Haddad et al. 2000; Anderson et al. 2008; Jones and Huo 2006).

However, the prosthesis used as spacer is expensive and discarded after six weeks. The surgical treatment is twice as expensive as that of an aseptic revision and 3 to 4 times that of a primary TKA. Much of that cost was due to the prolonged hospitalization (Haddad et al. 2000).

The PROSTALAC spacer showed acceptable infection eradication with a reasonable ROM between stages (Haddad et al. 2000), but concerns of mechanical complications, extra costs and increased operative time have been raised (Cuckler 2005; Anderson et al. 2008).

Controversy still exists regarding the use of the original autoclaved femoral component as articulating spacer as described by Hofmann et al. (Anderson et al. 2008).

A concern with any interim spacer technique is retention of foreign material within the joint. It would seem that a temporary articulating system made of only AB cement would have theoretical advantages over those with metal and plastic. *Kendall et al.* (1995) reported that Staphylococcus aureus and epidermidis can be found viable on AB-impregnated PMMA disks after 96 hours of incubation in vitro. They subsequently reported the opposite in vivo. The implants used in the series of Hofmann et al. (1995, 2005) and Masri et al. (1998) were metal and plastic implants. The similarly low infection rate despite metal and plas-

tic parts may be related to the high-dose AB used in the cement (Fehring et al. 2000).

Few studies have compared static (SS) and articular spacers (AS). *Fehring et al.* (2000) conducted a study to determine whether an AS could diminish bone loss, decrease operative time or improve function without a concomitant increase in infection rate compared to a static. They found no significance in the reinfection rate. It was encouraging to see that allowing some ROM did not lead to an increased reinfection rate. On the other hand, they were disappointed to see that function and ROM were not significantly different between both groups. It has to be noted that patient treated with an AS were immobilized for 10 days postoperatively. The authors suggested that more aggressive formal physical therapy could improve eventual function. This is, however, not without risks.

Some authors think that resting the joint is an important part of treatment for a septic joint and that aggressive ROM should be delayed until the infection is well under control (Fehring et al. 2000). On the other hand, excellent results were reported in studies were the rehabilitation protocol advised active mobilization directly postoperatively, continuous passive motion and full weight-bearing as tolerated (Meek et al. 2004; Cuckler 2005; Anderson et al. 2008).

Emerson et al. (2002) found their hypothesis to be true, finding significantly better knee flexion in patients with mobile spacers versus static spacers with no evidence for a higher complication or infection rate. They did show a more difficult removal and surgical time at re-implantation of the articulating spacers. Because of the late stage recurrence of infection, it is apparent that patients with infected TKA need long-term FU after treatment.

Freeman et al. (2007) could only find a significant difference in the percentage good to excellent functional results of AS versus SS.

There has been a general assumption that the outcome for septic revision is worse. Data provided by Meek et al. (2004) suggest that this is not necessarily so. They compared the functional results of 111 revisions, 54 of septic causes, 57 aseptic. The infected TKA were treated with a PROSTALAC mobile articulating spacer. At a mean of 41 months, none of the outcomes were significantly worse for the septic group.

Another study reported the opposite showing that results of revision for infected TKA are not as good as results for revision for any other reason (Barrack et al. 2000).

Conclusion

Two-stage re-implantation has become the gold standard for treating patients presenting with a chronic infection after total knee arthroplasty.

A first stage with thorough debridement of soft tissues, removal of all components and cement and implantation of an antibiotic-impregnated spacer is the first step. It should be followed by a minimum inverval period of 6 weeks during which intravenous antibiotics are given based on cultures and sensitivity of the infecting organism(s). A second stage re-implantation can then be carried out when the infection is eradicated, based on a combination of clinical examination, laboratory results (ESR, CRP, CBC), intraoperative cultures and optional a reaspiration.

Both static spacer blocks and articulating spacers have been used during the interval in between the two stages. There is a growing trend towards the use of articulating spacers in favor of the static spacers. The former allow weight-bearing, provide functional range of motion during the antibiotic therapy and maintain the bone-stock quality whereas the latter have the risk of stiffening of the knee joint, compromising the bone stock, necessitating a more aggressive surgical exposure at second-stage surgery and carry a greater risk for severe complications.

Up to today, all the published results lack significance to prove the superiority of articulating spacers over static spacers on functional scores, re-infection rates or pain outcome. Although articulating spacers have similar eradication rates compared to static spacers, small sample size, short FU and limited outcome measures have failed to confirm that patients have better long-term function if interim articulating spacers are used (Fehring et al. 2000; Wilde and Ruth 1988). In fact, articulating devices seem to have no functional advantage over static spacers but seem to facilitate re-implantation without an increase in rate of infection (Fehring et al. 2000).

There is, however, a statistically significant difference in postoperative range of motion, a minimal bone loss and a trend towards a significantly better functional outcome for articulating spacers.

The promising results with articulating spacers, without the complications of the static spacers need to be validated in future research.

The question still remains if an articulating spacer has the ability to combine all the advantages of a static spacer in eradicating deep infection after TKA and add a statistically significant improvement on functional outcome, in a cost-effective manner and on long-term follow-up.

References

Anderson JA, Sculco PK, Heitkemper S, Mayman DJ, Bostrom MP, Sculco TP (2009) An articulating spacer to treat and mobilize patients with infected total knee arthroplasty. J Arthroplasty 24(4): 631–5

Barrack RL, Engh G, Rorabeck C, Sawhney J, Woolfrey M (2000) Patient satisfaction and outcome after septic versus aseptic revision total knee arthroplasty. J Arthroplasty 15: 990–993

Bengtson K, Knutson K, Lidgren L (1986) Revision of infected knee arthroplasty. Acta Orthop Scand 57: 489–494

Bengtson S, Knutson K (1991) The infected knee arthroplasty: a 6-year follow-up of 357 cases. Acta Orthop Scand 62: 301–311

Booth RE Jr, Lotke PA (1989) The results of spacer block technique in revision of infected total knee arthroplasty. Clin Orthop Relat Res 248: 57–60

Borden LS, Gearen PF (1987) Infected total knee arthroplasty: a protocol for management. J Arthroplasty 2: 27–36

Buechel FF (1990) A sequential three-step lateral release for correcting fixed valgus knee deformities during total knee arthroplasty. Clin Orthop Relat Res 260: 170–5

Buechel FF, Femino FP, D'Alessio J (2004) Primary exchange revision arthroplasty for infected total knee replacement: a long-term study. Am J Orthop 33: 190 [discussion 198]

Burger RR, Basch T, Hopson CN (1991) Implant salvage in infected total knee arthroplasty. Clin Orthop Relat Res 273: 105–112

Calton TF, Fehring TK, Griffin WL (1997) Bone loss associated with the use of spacer blocks in infected total knee arthroplasty. Clin Orthop Relat Res 345: 148–154

Cohen JC, Hozak WJ, Cuckler JM, Booth RE (1988) Two-stage reimplantation of septic total knee arthroplasty. J Arthroplasty 3: 369–377

Cuckler JM (2005) The infected total knee: management options. J Arthroplasty 20 (Suppl 2): 33–36

Emerson RH Jr, Muncie M, Tarbox TR, Higgins LL (2002) Comparison of a static with a mobile spacer in total knee infection. Clin Orthop Relat Res 404: 132–138

Falahee MH, Matthews LS, Kaufer H (1987) Resection arthroplasty as a salvage procedure for a knee with infection after a total arthroplasty. J Bone Joint Surg 69: 1013–1021

Fehring TK, Odum S, Calton TF, Mason JB (2000) Articulating versus static spacers in revision total knee arthroplasty for sepsis. The Ranawat Award. Clin Orthop Relat Res 380: 9–16

Freeman MA, Sudlow RA, Casewell MW, Radcliff SS (1985) The management of infected total knee replacements. J Bone Joint Surg 67: 764–768

Freeman MG, Fehring TK, Odum SM, Fehring K, Griffin WL, Mason JB (2007) Functional advantage of articulating versus static spacers in 2-stage revision for total knee arthroplasty infection. J Arthroplasty 22: 1116–1121

Gill GS, Mills DM (1991) Long-term follow-up evaluation of 1000 consecutive cemented total knee arthroplasties. Clin Orthop 273: 66–76

Göksan SB, Freeman MA (1992) One-stage reimplantation for infected total knee arthroplasty. J Bone Joint Surg Br 74: 78–82

Goldberg VM, Figgie MP, Figgie III HE, Sobel M (1988) The results of revision total knee arthroplasty. Clin Orthop Relat Res 226: 86–92

Grogan TJ, Dorey F, Rollins J, Amstutz HC (1986) Deep sepsis following total knee arthroplasty. Ten-year experience at the University of California at Los Angeles Medical Center. J Bone Joint Surg 68: 226–234

Haddad FS, Masri BA, Campbell D, McGraw RW, Beauchamp CP, Duncan CP (2000) The PROSTALAC functional spacer in two-stage revision for infected knee replacements. Prosthesis of antibiotic-loaded acrylic cement. J Bone Joint Surg Br 82: 807–812

Haleem AA, Berry DJ, Hanssen AD (2004) Mid-term to long-term followup of two-stage reimplantation for infected total knee arthroplasty. Clin Orthop Relat Res 428: 35–39

Hartman MB, Fehring TK, Jordan L, Norton HJ (1991) Periprosthetic knee sepsis. Clin Orthop Relat Res 273: 113–118

Hirakawa K, Stulberg BN, Wilde AH, Bauer TW, Secic M (1998) Results of 2-stage reimplantation for infected total knee arthroplasty. J Arthroplasty 13: 22–28

Hofmann AA, Goldberg T, Tanner AM, Kurtin SM (2005) Treatment of infected total knee arthroplasty using an articulating spacer: 2- to 12-year experience. Clin Orthop Relat Res 430: 125–131

Hofmann AA, Kane KR, Tkach TK, Plaster RL, Camargo MP (1995) Treatment of infected total knee arthroplasty using an articulating spacer. Clin Orthop Relat Res 321: 45–54

Insall JN, Thompson FM, Brause BD (1983) Two-stage reimplantation for the salvage of infected total knee arthroplasty. J Bone Joint Surg Am 65: 1087–1098

Johnson DP, Bannister GC (1986) The outcome of infected arthroplasty of the knee. J Bone Joint Surg 68: 289–291

Jones RE, Huo MH (2006) The infected knee: all my troubles now. J Arthroplasty 21 (Suppl 1): 50–53

Kaufer H, Matthews LS (1986) Resection arthroplasty: An alternative to arthrodesis for salvage of the infected total knee arthroplasty. Instructional Course Lectures 35: 283–289

Kendall RW, Duncan CP, Beauchamp CP (1995) Bacterial growth on antibiotic-loaded acrylic cement. A prospective in vivo retrieval study. J Arthroplasty 10: 817–822

Laskin RS (1976) Modular total knee-replacement arthroplasty: A review of eighty-nine patients. J Bone Joint Surg Am 58: 766–773

Marsch PK, Cotler JM (1981) Management of an anaerobic infection in a prosthetic knee with long-term antibiotics alone: a case report. Clin Orthop Relat Res 155: 133–155

Mason JB, Fehring TK, Odum SM et al. (2003) The value of white blood cell counts before revision total knee arthroplasty. J Arthroplasty 18: 1038–1043

Masri BA, Duncan CP, Beauchamp CP (1998) Long-term elution of antibiotics from bone-cement: an in vivo study using the prosthesis of antibiotic-loaded acrylic cement (PROSTALAC) system. J Arthroplasty 13: 331–338

McPherson EJ, Patzakis MJ, Gross JE, Holtom PD, Song M, Dorr LD (1997) Infected total knee arthroplasty. Two-stage reimplantation with a gastrocnemius rotational flap. Clin Orthop Relat Res 341: 73–81

Meek RM, Dunlop D, Garbuz DS, McGraw R, Greidanus NV, Masri BA (2004) Patient satisfaction and functional status after aseptic versus septic revision total knee arthroplasty using the PROSTALAC articulating spacer. J Arthroplasty 19: 874–879

Morrey BF, Westholm F, Schoifet S, Rand JA, Bryan RS (1989) Long-term results of various treatment options for infected total knee arthroplasty. Clin Orthop Relat Res 248: 120–128

Petty W, Bryan RS, Coventry MB, Peterson LF (1975) Infection after total knee arthroplasty. Orthop Clin North Am 6: 1005–1014

Rand JA, Bryan RS, Morrey BF, Westholm F (1986) Management of infected total knee arthroplasty. Clin Orthop Relat Res 205: 75–85

Rand JA, Fitzgerald RH Jr (1989) Diagnosis and management of the infected total knee arthroplasty. Orthop Clin North Am 20: 201–210

Rosenberg AG, Haas B, Barden R, Marquez D, Landon GC, Galante JO (1988) Salvage of infected total knee arthroplasty. Clin Orthop Rel Res 226: 29–33

Schoicet JD, Morrey BF (1990) Treatment of infection after Total knee arthroplasty by debridement with retention of the components. J Bone Joint Surg Am 72: 1383–1390

Teeny SM, Dorr L, Murata G, Conaty P (1990) Treatment of infected total knee arthroplasty. Irrigation and debridement versus two-stage reimplantation. J Arthroplasty 5: 35–39

Tsukayama DT, Goldberg VM, Kyle R (2003) Diagnosis and management of infection after total knee arthroplasty. J Bone Joint Am 85-A (Suppl 1): S75–80

Walker RH, Schurman DJ (1984) Management of infected total knee arthroplasties. Clin Orthop Relat Res 186: 81–89

Wilde AH, Ruth JT (1988) Two-stage reimplantation in infected total knee arthroplasty. Clin Orthop Relat Res 236: 23–25

Windsor RE, Insall JN, Urs WK, Miller DV, Brause BD (1990) Two stage reimplantation for the salvage of total knee arthroplasty complicated by infection. Further follow-up and refinement of indications. J Bone Joint Surg Am 72: 272–278

Woods GW, Lionberger DR, Tullos HS (1983) Failed total knee arthroplasty: revision and arthrodesis for infection and non-infectious complications. Clin Orthop Relat Res 173: 184–190

Spacer Management in Periprosthetic Infections

Christian Eberhardt

Introduction

In 1890 Themistokles Gluck, a German surgeon, was the first who implanted an endoprosthesis made from ivory into a human joint. Unfortunately, this event was also the beginning of history of periprosthetic infections because Gluck selected a knee joint destroyed by infection from tuberculosis.

Infection rates in modern hip and knee arthroplasty ranges from 1 to 2%. Recently Peersman et al. (2002) reported a deep infection rate in total knee arthroplasty of 0.43% in a series of 6439 consecutive patients under strong antiseptic prophylaxis including use of vertical laminar air flow and body exhaust suits. This is encouraging but, however, periprosthetic infection is still a complication of major concern and a devastating problem. Many of those cases require removal of the infected implant. This can be managed by one- or two-stage revision. One-stage revision is advocated by only a limited number of authors, two-stage revision is widely accepted and success rates at around 90% have been reported. The main problem in case of a two-stage strategy is the time between the stages.

Of course, the most important goal is control and eradication of infection. The first procedure that demonstrated potency for sufficient elimination of infection was resection arthroplasty

(■ Fig. 9.1). Unfortunately, you have to accept functional disadvantages like limb shortening, soft-tissue retraction, ligament contracture, tissue adherence, arthrofibrosis, extensor lag, quadriceps

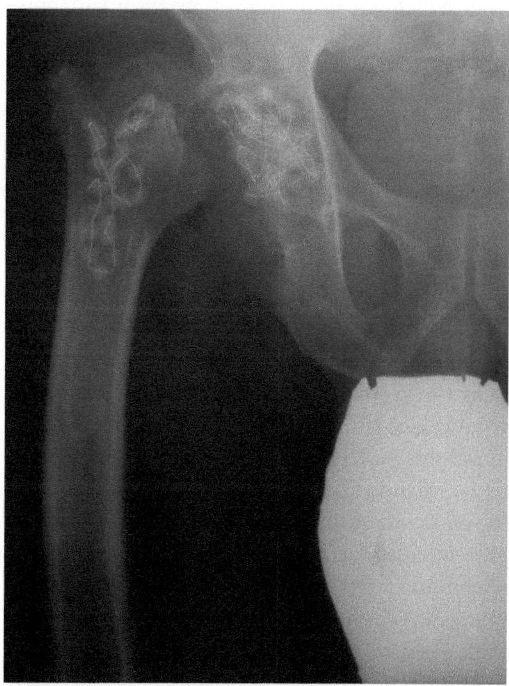

■ **Fig. 9.1.** Resection arthroplasty (Girdlestone situation) after infected total hip arthroplasty

shortening, disuse osteoporosis and bone resorption. This leads to a difficult exposure at the second-stage surgery, often resulting in numerous complications and unsatisfied or poor functional results.

Non-Articulating Spacers

To overcome these problems temporary spacers had been introduced. As a first edition of a spacer the non-articulating (block, static) spacer was invented initially by Cohan et al. in 1988 for infected total knee arthroplasty (Fig. 9.2). It was a handmade polymethylmetacrylate (PMMA) cement block impregnated with one or more antibiotics for high local antibiotic concentrations at the infected site and fashioned to fit the bone stock defect. Advantages compared to resection arthroplasty were the possibility of preserving limb length and prevention of soft-tissue retraction. Anyway, joint movement was still impossible and cast immobilization often required. Furthermore a wide variety of disadvantages concerning soft tissue (ligament contracture, tissue adherence, arthrofibrosis, extensor lag), bone tissue (bone erosion caused by spacer shifting, disuse osteoporosis) and the spacer itself like spacer dislocation (Fig. 9.3) or spacer fracture remained unsolved. Anyway there is still need for the use of static spacers at least in cases of severe bone loss or difficult infection control (Case Report no. 1)

Case Report 1: Treatment with a Non-Articulating Spacer in Infected Total Knee Arthroplasty and Severe Bone Loss

An 80-year old male had clinical and radiographic signs (Fig. 9.4a,b) of chronic infection after total arthroplasty of the right knee in 2004. Implant removal was performed in August 2008. Intraoperatively, extended bone loss of the femoral condylar region was detected, resulting in resection of metaphyseal condylar region. Decision was made for a temporary replacement with a non-articulating spacer (Fig. 9.4c,d), after 6 weeks and clinical infection control reconstruction with re-implantation of a constraint condylar replacement (Fig. 9.4e,f) under use of commercially antibiotic laden cement finished the two-stage procedure.

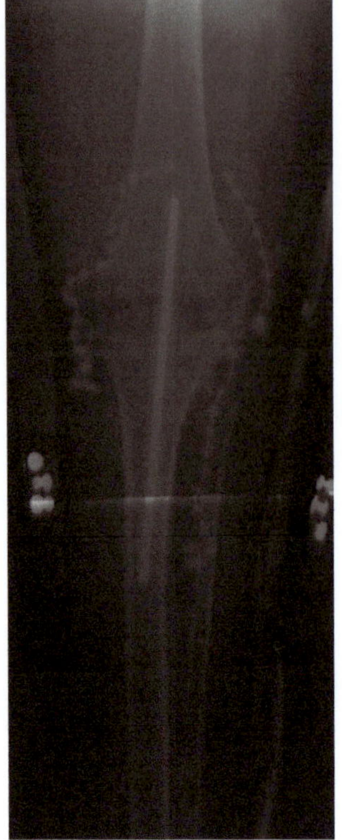

Fig. 9.2. Non-articulating spacer after infected total knee arthroplasty with additional antibiotic beads

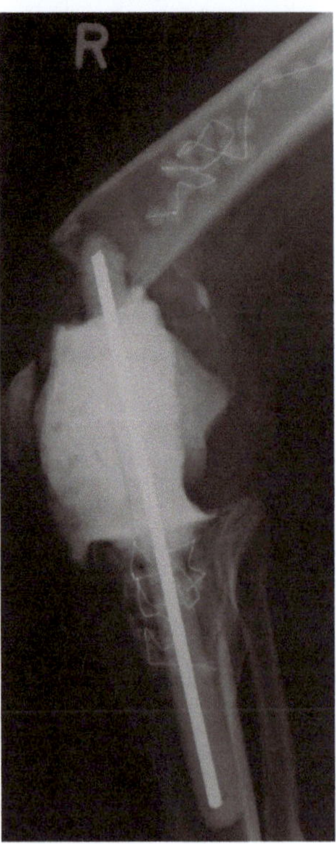

Fig. 9.3. Dislocation of a non-articulating knee spacer

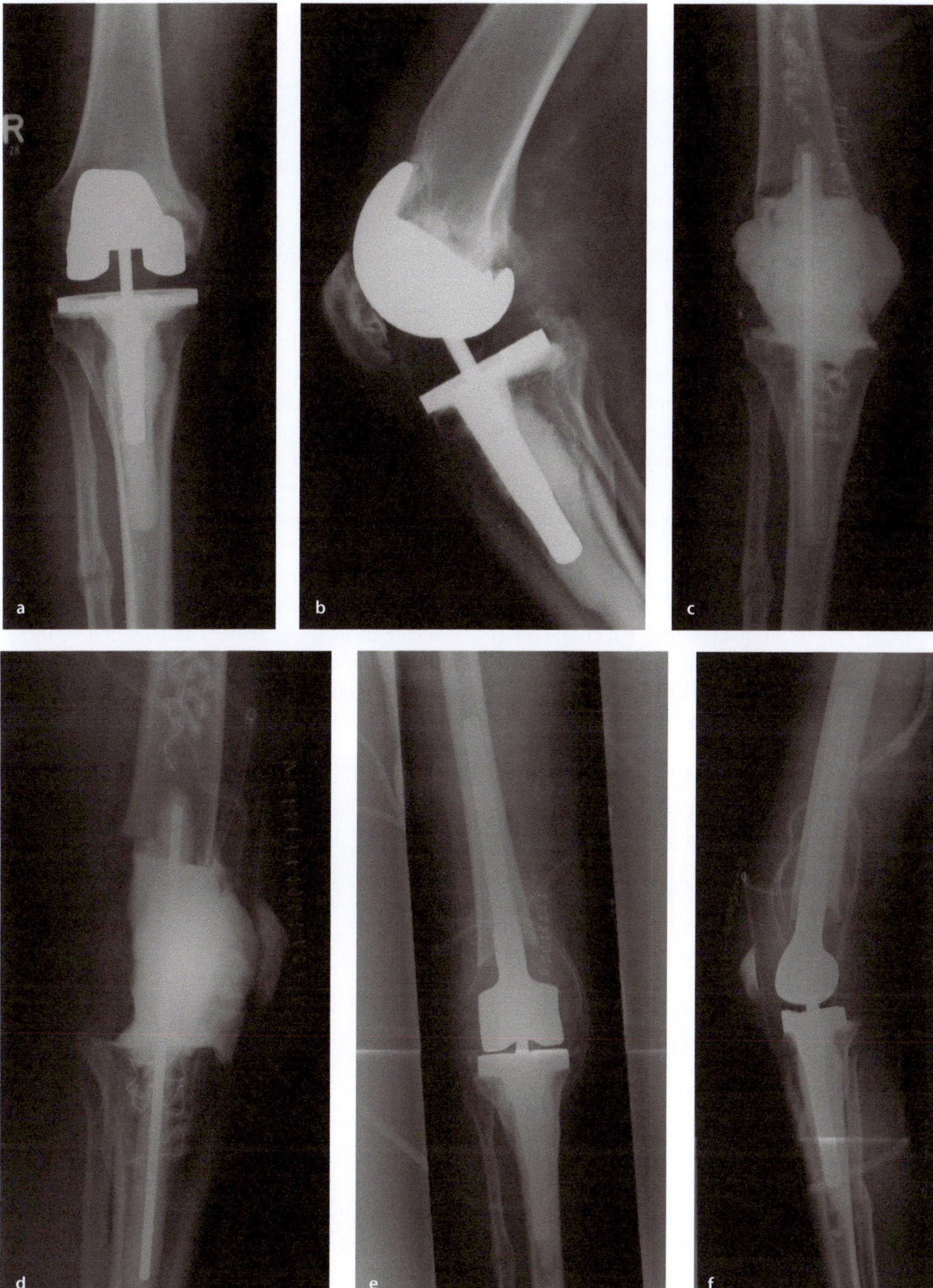

Fig. 9.4. a,b Radiographs (a.p., lateral) after total knee arthroplasty and osteolysis of the medial and lateral femoral condyle related to chronic periprosthetic infection. **c,d** Radiographs (a.p., lateral) of a temporary replacement with a static spacer. **e,f** Radiographs (a.p., lateral) after second stage re-implantation with constraint condylar replacement

Articulating Spacers

Spacer Prosthesis

Optimizing the functional outcome without compromising the security regarding infection control was the scope of further developments, resulting in the introduction of articulating (mobile) spacers. The so-called spacer prosthesis was the first edition of an articulating spacer. It was simply the removed and cleaned infected implant that was re-sterilized in an autoclave and re-implanted between the stages. Temporary fixation to the bone was achieved with the use antibiotic-laden cement applied at the end of its working phase. This technique enabled an easy removal of the spacer at second-stage surgery without additional bone loss. Partial weight-bearing and unlimited range of motion were encouraged for the duration of spacer treatment and second-stage surgery was planned after infection control.

Using this technique, Wentworth et al. (2002) reported about 135 patients with infected total hip arthroplasty. Persisting infections and recurrence rate were both at 8.8%, most important complications were femur fractures in 12.6% and spacer dislocations in 8.1%. Hofmann et al. (2005) reported about 27 patients using antibiotic bone cement laden with 4.8 g tobramycin to 40 g cement, followed by systemic antibiotic therapy for 6 weeks. They had a recurrence rate of 4% after 76 months, one femur fracture and a dislocation rate of 14.8%. With infected total knee arthroplasty Emerson et al. (2002) had a mean follow-up of 36 month in 22 patients and a recurrence rate of 9% under the use of 3.6 g tobramycin and 2 g vancomycin to 40 g cement. Better results came from Hofmann et al. (1995) with no recurrence after 30-month follow-up. Anyway, the use of spacer prosthesis can interfere with national regulations because in some countries it is not allowed to re-implant an infected, cleaned and re-sterilized implant. The main argument against this technique is the presence of metal and polyethylene components between the stages and the assumption that these foreign body materials could be the reason for persistence or later recurrence of infection.

All PMMA Spacers

To overcome these concerns, mobile spacers completely made from antibiotic-laden PMMA cement were established. One possibility is a handmade preparation (■ Fig. 9.5), another is the use of intraoperatively prepared molds from the removed implant. An early report in this technique was given by Goldstein et al. (2001) who described the intraoperative manufacturing in revision of infected total knee arthroplasty. It is a convenient procedure in total knee arthroplasty, the shape and size of the spacer is close to the removed implant, it is cost-effective but time-consuming. As far as time in the operation unit is very expensive, there is an argument for commercially prepared molds (■ Fig. 9.6a,b). This technique is also convenient for total hip arthroplasty but causes additional costs. The latest evolution of mobile spacers is a commercially preformed spacer for infected total knee and hip arthroplasty (■ Fig. 9.7a,b) which is available in different sizes. The handling of these devices is quite comfortable and time-saving with an easy storage system.

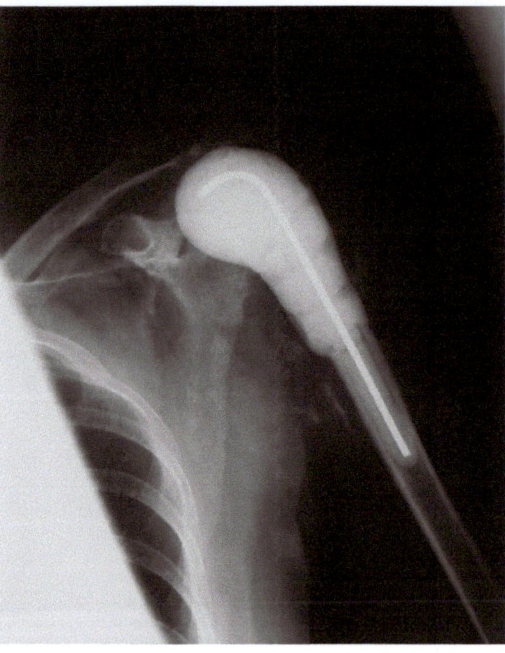

■ **Fig. 9.5.** Handmade all PMMA spacer of the proximal humerus

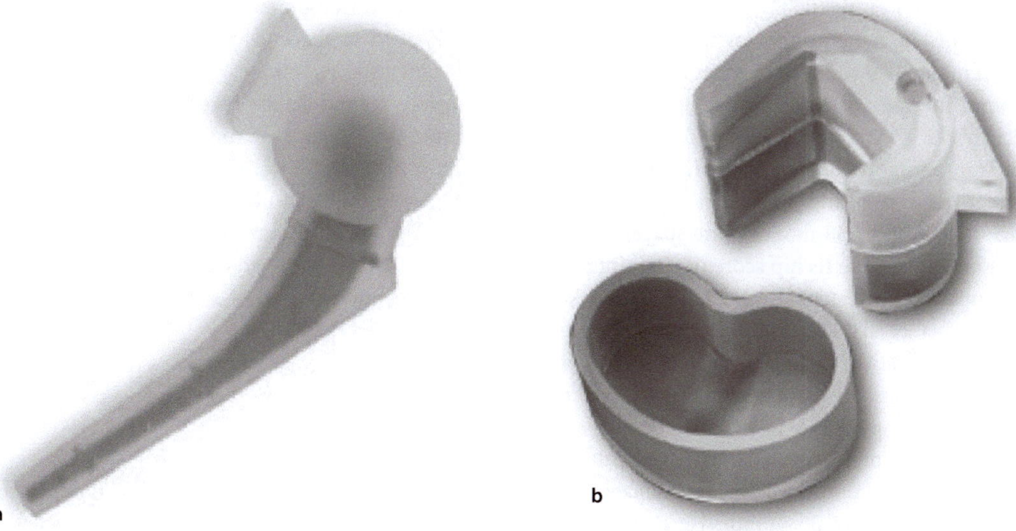

Fig. 9.6. a Commercially prepared spacer mold for total hip arthroplasty. **b** Commercially prepared spacer mold for total knee arthroplasty

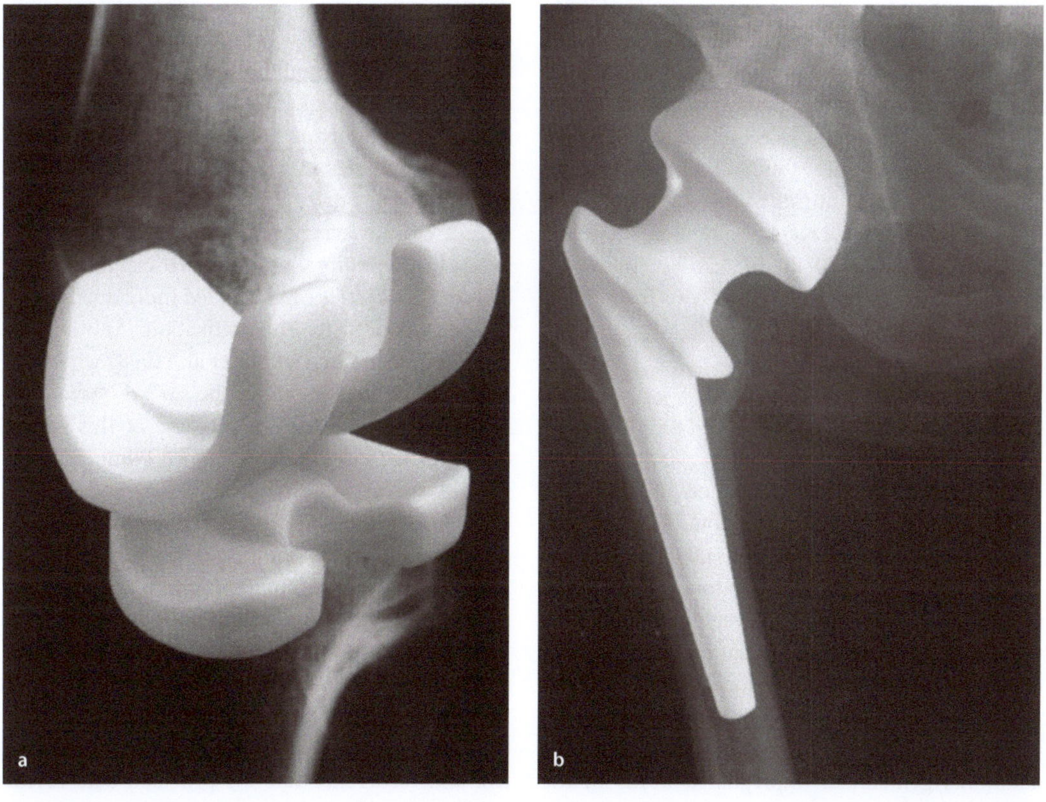

Fig. 9.7. a Commercially preformed PMMA spacer for infected total knee arthroplasty. **b** Commercially preformed PMMA spacer for infected total hip arthroplasty

Yamamoto et al. (2003) presented a series of 17 patients in management of infected total hip replacement. They added 0.5 g gentamicin to 40 g cement, in cases of MRSA infections 1 g gentamicin and 2 g vancomycin were added, followed by systemic antibiotic application. He had infection control in all cases and no recurrence after an average follow-up of 38 month. One spacer dislocation and a mean Harris hip score of 89 points were documented. For revision total knee arthroplasty Drubhakula et al. (2004) reported a consecutive series of 24 patients using 2.4 g tobramycin and 1 g vancomycin to 40 g cement with systemic antibiotic therapy for 6 weeks. After an average interim period of 12 weeks he achieved infection control in 92% and noticed no recurrence over an average follow-up of 33 month. He had two persistent infections (8%) with MRSA that required above-knee amputation after multiple revisions, the average knee flexion was 104°, the average Special Surgery Knee Score 82 points at latest follow-up. Similar results were given by Ha (2006) in a series of 12 consecutive patients. They added 4.8 g tobramycin and 4 g vancomycin to 40 g cement and did not mention any systemic antibiotic therapy. After an average interim period of 9 weeks infection control in all cases was achieved and no recurrence occurred during follow-up period from 2–3.5 years. The average knee flexion increased from preoperatively 79° to 102° at last follow-up, the average Knee Society Knee Score from 30 to 87 points.

Case Report 2: Treatment with an Articulating Spacer in Infected Total Knee Arthroplasty

A 71-year old female complained of persisting knee pain for 3 months after total knee arthroplasty 2 years before. She had no clinical signs of infection and regular laboratory values (ESR, CRP, WBC). Radiographs revealed osteolysis at the medial and lateral tibial plateau (Fig. 9.8a,b), after joint aspiration Staphylococcus aureus was cultured. The implant was removed and replaced by a commercially preformed mobile spacer with additional gentamicin impregnated beads in the femoral and tibial canal to enhance local antibiotic concentration (Fig. 9.8c,d). Fixation was achieved with the use of commercially antibiotic-laden cement applied at the end of its working phase in poor cementing technique. After infection control and before second-stage procedure the knee demonstrated good range of motion with extension/flexion 0°/0°/100° (Fig. 9.8e). As a result of first-stage cementing technique the spacer could be removed at second-stage without any additional bone loss (Fig. 9.8f,g) and reconstruction was finished by re-implantation of a constraint total knee arthroplasty (Fig. 9.8h,i).

Concerns

Despite the promising clinical results, there have been still several concerns in the use of temporary spacers. One important issue is elution characteristics. Especially the commercially preformed spacers were accused to compromise the individual choice and dosage of antibiotics, furthermore, there were discussions about a possible deterioration of release kinetics due to the fabrication process under high pressure. Addressing these concerns, Bertazzoni et al. (2004) could show that at time of explantation 3–6 months after implantation these spacers still provide a sufficient antibiotic release. Furthermore, additional antibiotic release can be achieved by the use of antibiotic beads in the femoral and/or tibial canal, culture-directed antibiotics can be added individually with the cement used for spacer fixation. Another remark was made by Holtom et al. (1998) who pronounced the importance of the surface-to-volume ratio and showed that an increase of this ration enhances the release in vancomycin-impregnated PMMA spacers. Greene et al. (1998) and Penner et al. (1996) focused on different release rates of different antibiotics showing a higher release of tobramycin compared to vancomycin and different release rates with different antibiotic combinations. Furthermore they described different elution rates from different cement brands with a better release from Palacos compared to Simplex cement. Going back to the clinical results regarding infection control and recurrence rate the provided data reveal good to excellent results proofing high sufficiency for this most important goal of treatment.

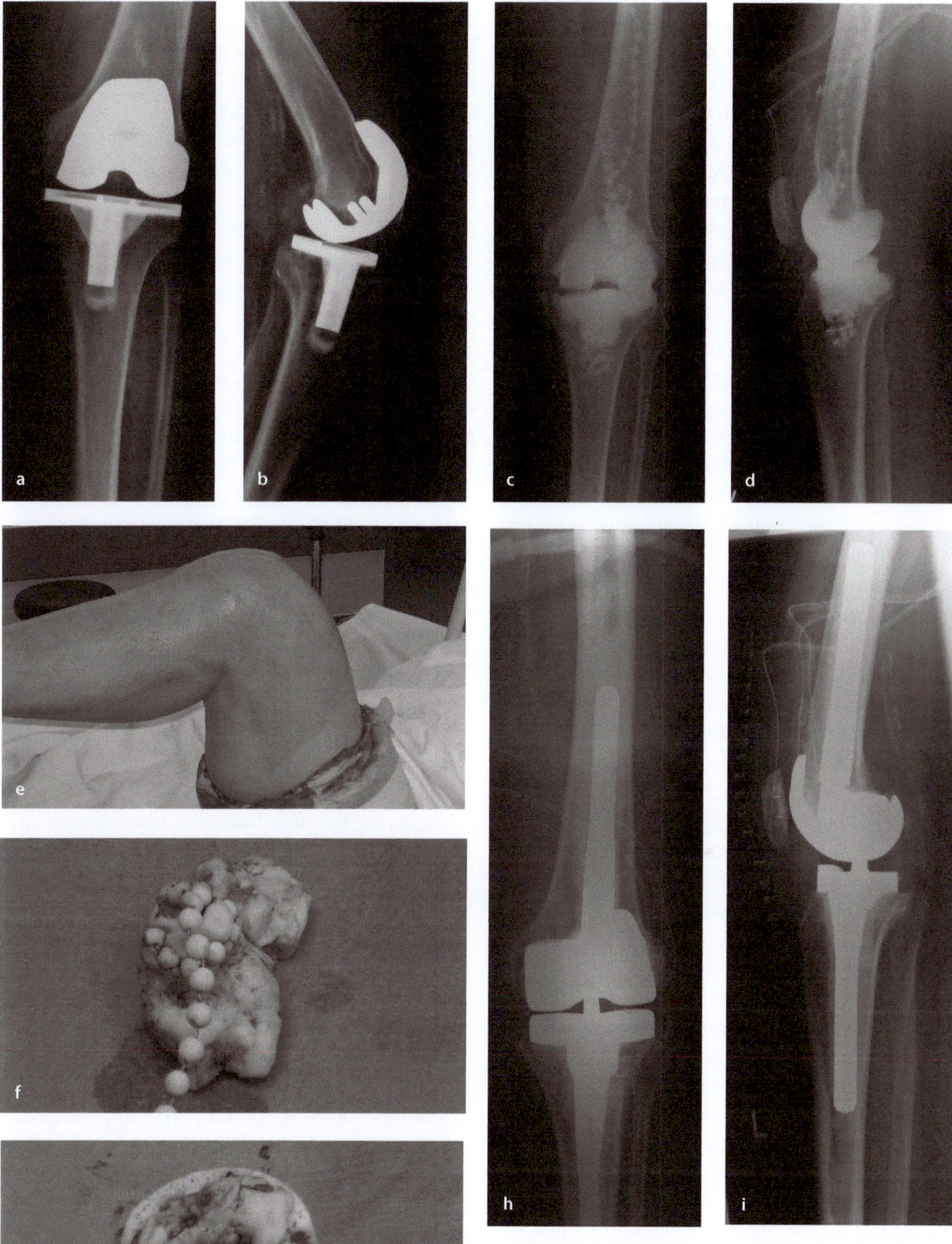

Fig. 9.8. a,b Radiographs (a.p., lateral) after total knee arthroplasty and osteolysis under tibial component related to periprosthetic infection. **c,d** Radiographs (a.p., lateral) after placement of a temporary mobile spacer. **e** Flexion capacity before second stage surgery. **f,g** Tibial and femoral spacer component after removal at second stage. **h,i** Second stage reconstruction with a constraint total knee arthroplasty

Another important issue is mechanical stability. Schöllner et al. (2003) reported about stability tests using an axial strength test and had failure loads around 1.6 kN. Inserted K-wires did not improve mechanical stability but prevented dislocation of the fragments. Similar tests were done by Kelm et al. (2001), in contrast they found failure loads around 20 kN. Finally, there is still discussion on the study protocol because axial strength tests do not represent the in-vivo loads of those spacers, so the clinical validity of these results remains unclear. Levin (1975) and Murray (1984) pointed out the importance of proportional weights of antibiotics added to the cement. Most surgeons accept an additive up to 10% of the used bone cement mass but recently Hsieh et al. (2005) used a mixture containing 20% of bone cement mass and noticed no signs of mechanical insufficiency of their spacers. Affatato et al. (2003) and Baleani et al. (2003) focused on wear debris and could show that it is depending on the spacer area. Anyway they concluded that partial weight-bearing of these spacers can be allowed because debris can be removed completely during second-stage surgery. Summarizing clinical results concerning the issue of mechanical stability, there are low rates of spacer fractures mostly associated with use of intraoperatively prepared hip spacers or/and incompliance with weight bearing. Reports on severe wear debris are only isolated, so there are no relevant problems with mechanical stability resulting in clinical consequences at least with the commercially preformed spacers.

Systemic safety is another important topic, in 2002 van Raaij et al. presented a case report about a 83-year old female with no history of kidney disease who suffered from renal failure after implantation of a 2 g gentamicin spacer with 7 additional chains of 30 gentamicin beads. Probably the side effects in this case report are related to the excessive use of cement beads because it is well known that release from those beads is up to 6-fold higher than from spacers (Moojen et al. 2008). Springer et al. (2004) designed a prospective study including 34 patients with a mean age of 66.5 years, half of them with risk factors for renal insufficiency. They constantly monitored the lab values including blood count, creatinine and liver function. A high impregnation with 4 g vancomycin and 4.8 g gentamicin to 40 g cement was chosen, the average total dose per spacer was 10.5 g vancomycin and 12.5 g gentamicin. They noticed only one transient serum creatinine rise at the first day after operation that completely recovered until the third day and no other side effects like hypersensitivity or allergy. The recurrence rate at latest follow-up was 8%. Reports of severe systemic side effects are rare and often not clearly related to the use of a spacer, so in conclusion spacers provide high systemic safety.

A last concern with growing importance in our time is costs of spacer treatment. Using commercially preformed spacers you have to deal with additional € 1000.– plus the cost for cement for fixation and antibiotics. If you prefer commercially preformed molds you lower your costs but intraoperative preparation time is expanded. Adding up the costs of this additional time ends in a total very close to the costs of treatment with preformed spacers. Conclusion in this issue is well known: Septic surgery is expensive.

Advantages of Mobile Spacers

Considering the high treatment costs there is still controversy on the potential benefit of mobile spacers. In the literature there are only few reports on direct comparisons between mobile spacers versus static spacers or resection arthroplasty. For management of infected total hip replacement Hsieh et al. (2004) presented a comparison of resection arthroplasty with antibiotic beads versus mobile spacer in a consecutive series of 143 patients. They were able to include 128 patients, with an average follow-up of 4.9 years. 70 patients received resection arthroplasty, 58 spacer treatment. Systemic antibiotic therapy was applied for at least 2 weeks and between the two groups no statistical differences regarding age, follow-up, re-implantation technique, preoperative hip score, first-stage details and duration of interim period were evaluated. Group comparison revealed significant advantages for the spacer group during second-stage procedure regarding operative time, blood loss, transfusion units and duration of hospital stay and no differences in security expressed by infection control and recurrence rate (▣ Table 9.1a). Interim hip score revealed a significant advantage for the spacer group while the hip score at latest follow-up was equal to the resection group. The dislocation rate after second stage re-implantation was significantly lower in the spacer group (▣ Table 9.1b). In summary, the authors recommended the use of mobile spacers due to their advantages at second-stage surgery and the considerable reduced dislocation rate. In revision total knee arthroplasty Fehring et al. (2000) reported excellent results in infection control for both mobile and static spacers, a recurrence rate of 12% for static and 7%

for mobile spacers and a facilitation of second stage surgery with mobile spacers. Postoperative range of motion showed a tendency towards better results in the mobile spacer group (105° vs. 98°) without statistical significance. They detected problems with severe bone loss in the static spacer group related to a prolonged interim period (mean 48 days without bone loss, mean 88 days with bone loss). Defects were more pronounced on the femoral side (average 12.8 mm) than on the tibial side (average 6.2 mm). Emerson et al. (2002) presented even better results in 26 patients with static and 22 with mobile spacers. They added 3.6 g tobramycin and 2 g vancomycin to 40 g cement followed by systemic antibiotic therapy for at least 6 weeks and an interim of 6–12 weeks with partial weight-bearing. One static spacer subluxation was noticed and bone loss »did not seem to be a problem« in this study. After a mean follow-up of 3.6 years recurrence rate was equal in both groups but the mobile group revealed significantly higher range of motion (▣ Table 9.2).

Conclusion

A final consideration of the present literature on spacers is difficult. There are varying study designs, most studies include only a limited number of patients and mostly provide only medium term of follow-up. There is no common standard in revision surgery of periprosthetic infections, there are different surgical techniques, different techniques in spacer preparation and different antibiotic loading doses for spacer impregnation. Furthermore, the postoperative treatment provides great variations especially in important parameters like dosage and duration of postoperative antibiotic regiment or duration of interim period. A standard definition of the terms infection control and recurrence rate, the two most important parameters of treatment success is not existing so far. This leads us to a database that is very heterogeneous and in parts inconsistent and therefore a comparison of the results of present literature is quite difficult and often impossible.

Despite these problems there are a few statements that can be made finally. There are still

▣ **Table 9.1a.** Intergroup comparison (Hsieh et al. 2004)

	Resection	Spacer	P
2nd, operative time	205 min	129	*
2nd, blood loss	2033 ml	952 ml	*
2nd, transfusion	3.7 units	1.4 units	*
2nd, hospital stay	24.8 d	18.3 d	*
Infection recurrence	1.6%	1.8%	
Infection control over all	94.3%	96.5%	

▣ **Table 9.1b.** Intergroup comparison (Hsieh et al. 2004)

	Resection	Spacer	P
Interim hip score	10.2	13.3	*
Late FU hip score	15.3	15.8	
Post OP dislocation	14.3%	1.8%	*

▣ **Table 9.2.** Intergroup comparison (Emerson et al. 2002)

	Static	Mobile	P
Infection control	100%	100%	
Recurrence (3.6y)	7.6%	9.0%	
Flexion, preop	79.3°	73.4°	
Flexion, postop	93.7°	107.8°	*

concerns on the issue of mechanical stability regarding spacer fracture. Hip spacers seem to be more problematic, especially in cases of excessive loading due to incompliance with weight-bearing or adipositas. It remains unclear if inserted k-wires do have the potential to increase failure load. At least they prevent fragment dislocation, so in most cases a spacer fracture is without clinical consequences. Commercially preformed spacers appear to be superior to hand-made. Spacer dislocation is another urgent problem, especially with the use of hip spacer but even here clinical consequences are rare. Anyway, spacers provide high systemic safety and sufficient antibiotic release with good to excellent results in clinical outcome regarding infection control and recurrence rate. Static spacers are still a treatment option at least in cases of severe bone loss or difficult infection control. Mobile spacers demonstrate better results in preservation of bone stock, seem to facilitate re-implantation and appear to have advantages in functional outcome at least for short time follow-up.

In cases of a two-stage treatment of infected total joint arthroplasty the implantation of a temporary antibiotic laden spacer is currently the most commonly used method. Mobile spacers are first choice and should be used in all appropriate cases, static spacers should be chosen in those cases where mobile spacers for some reasons are not appropriate, resection arthroplasty with beads and no spacer should be the option for difficult selected cases representing the salvage procedure in septic orthopedic surgery.

References

Affatato S, Mattarozi A, Taddei P, Robotti P, Soffiatti R, Sudanese A, Toni A (2003) Investigations on the wear behaviour of temporary PMMA-based hip Spacer-G. Proc Inst Mech Eng 217: 1–8

Baleani M, Cristofolini L, Minari C, Toni A (2003) Fatigue strength of PMMA bone cement mixed with gentamicin and barium sulphate vs. pure PMMA. Proc Inst Mech Eng 217: 9–12

Bertazzoni E, Benini A, Magnan B, Bartolozzi P (2004) Release of gentamicin and vancomycin from temporary human hip spacers in two-stage revision of infected arthroplasty. J Antimicrob Chemother 53: 329–334

Cohen JC, Hozack W, Cuckler JM, Booth RE Jr (1988) Two-stage reimplantation of septic total knee arthroplasty. A report of three cases using an antibiotic-PMMA spacer block. J Arthroplasty 3: 369–377

Drubhakula SM, Czajka J, Fuchs MD, Uhl RL (2004) Antibiotic-loaded articulating cement spacer in the 2-stage exchange of infected total knee arthroplasty. J Arthroplasty 19: 768–774

Emerson RH, Muncie M, Tarbox TR, Higgins LL (2002) Comparison of a static with a mobile spacer in total knee infection. Clin Orthop 404: 132–138

Fehring TK, Odum S, Calton TF, Mason JB (2000) Articulating versus static spacers in revision total knee arthroplasty. Clin Orthop 380: 9–16

Goldstein WM, Kopplin M, Wall R, Berland K (2001) Temporary articulating methylmethacrylate antibiotic spacer. A new method of manufacturing a custom articulating spacer. J Bone Joint Surg 83A (Suppl 2): 92-97

Greene N, Holtom PD, Warren CA, Ressler RL, Shepherd L, MC Pherson EJ, Patzakis MJ (1998) In vitro elution of tobramycin and vancomycin polymethylmethacrylate beads and spacers from Palacos and Simplex. Am J Orthop 27: 201–205

Ha CW (2006) A technique for intraoperative construction of antibiotic spacers. Clin Orthop 445: 204–209

Hofmann AA, Goldberg TD, Tanner AM, Cook TM (2005) Ten-year experience using an articulating cement hip spacer for the treatment of chronically infected total hip. J Arthroplasty 20: 874–879

Hofmann AA, Kane KR, Tkach TK, Plaster RL, Camargo MP (1995) Treatment of infected total knee arthroplasty using an articulating spacer. Clin Orthop 321: 45–54

Holtom PD, Warren CA, Greene NW, Bravos PD, Ressler RL, Shepherd L, McPherson EJ, Patzakis MJ (1998) Relation of surface area to in vitro elution characteristics of vancomycin-impregnated polymethylmethacrylate spacers. Am J Orthop 27: 207–210

Hsieh PH, Shih CH, Chang YH, Lee MS, Shih HN, Yanh WE (2004) Two-stage revision hip arthroplasty for infection: comparison between the interim use of antibiotic-loaded cement beads and a spacer prosthesis. J Bone Joint Surg 86A: 1989–1997

Hsieh PH, Shih CH, Chang YH, Lee MS, Yanh WE, Shih HN (2005) Treatment of deep infection of the hip associated with massive bone loss. Two-stage revision with antibiotic-loaded interim cement prosthesis followed by reconstruction with allograft. J Bone Joint Surg 87B: 770–775

Kelm J, Regitz T, Schmitt E (2001) Infektsanierung durch resistenzgerechte Hüftinterimsprothese und Antibiotikakette. J DPGW 23: 61–62

Levin PD (1975) The effectiveness of various antibiotics in methylmethacrylate. J Bone Joint Surg 57B: 234–237

Moojen DJ Hentenaar B, Charles Vogely H, Verbout AJ, Castelein RM, Dhert WJ (2008) In vitro release of antibiotics from commercial PMMA beads and articulating hip spacers. J Arthroplasty 21: S0883–5403

Murray WR (1984) Use of antibiotic-containing bone cement. Clin Orthop 190: 89–95

Peersman G, Laskin R, Davis J, Peterson M (2002) Infection in total knee replacement: a retrospective review 6489 total knee replacements. Clin Ortho 392: 15–23

Penner MJ, Masri BA, Duncan CP (1996) Elution characteristics of vancomycin and tobramycin combined in acrylic bone cement. J Arthroplasty 11: 939–944

Schöllner C, Füderer S, Rompe JD, Eckhardt A (2003) Individual bone cement spacers for septic hip revision. Arch Orthop Trauma Surg 123: 254–259

Springer BD, Lee GC, Osmon D, Haidukewych GJ, Hanssen AD, Jacofsky DJ (2004) Systemic safety of high-dose antibiotic-loaded cement spacers after resection of an infected total knee arthroplasty. Clin Orthop 427: 47–51

van Raaij TM, Visser LE, Vulto AG, Verhaar JA (2002) Acute renal failure after local gentamicin treatment in an infected total knee arthroplasty. J Arthroplasty 17: 948–950

Wentworth SJ, Masri BA, Duncan CP, Southworth CB (2002) Hip prosthesis of antibiotic-loaded acrylic cement for the treatment of infections following total hip arthroplasty. J Bone Joint Surg 84A (Suppl 2): 123–128

Yamamoto K, Miyagawa N, Masaoka T, Katori Y, Shishido T, Imakiire A (2003) Clinical effectiveness of antibiotic-impregnated cement spacers for the treatment of infected implants of the hip joint. J Orthop Sci 8: 823–828

Observational Study of Bone Cement with Two Antibiotics in Revision Arthroplasty of Knee and Hip

Joachim Sauer

Participating physicians: Constantin Baumgarte, Kiel, Germany, Basilio José de la Torre, Guadalajara, Spain, Jürgen Esper, Nuremberg, Germany, Philipp Funovics, Vienna, Austria, Hrubina Maroš, Pelhřimov, Czech Republic, Matthias Kemmerer, Frankfurt/Main, Germany, Kozák Martin, Karviná-Ráj, Czech Republic, Andreas Kostka, Berlin, Germany, Wilfried Materna, Graz, Austria, Christian Melzer, Bad Düben, Germany, Molano Muñoz, Vitoria, Spain, Andreas Peters, Frankfurt/ Main, Germany, Martin Rieger, Bremen, Germany, Martin Stuhlinger, Reutlingen, Germany, Fernando Trell, Valdemoro, Spain

Introduction

The replacement of hip and knee joints has been a standard surgical procedure for decades. Around 1.3 million hip replacements and 1.0 million knee replacements are conducted annually worldwide, in Germany about 150,000 hip prostheses and around 100,000 knee prostheses are implanted (Bundesgeschäftsstelle Qualitätssicherung GGmbH 2006, 2007; The Institute for Orthopaedics 2008). Up to a few years ago, the life of an endoprosthesis frequently exceeded the life expectancy of the patient. However, demographic trends along with increasing life expectancy mean that revision arthroplasty is becoming more important (Sculco 1993). Thus in Sweden from 1995 to 2000 already around 8% of the hip total prostheses were revised and from 1995 to 2004 around 6% of the knee total prostheses (Kärrholm et al. 2007; Lidgren and Robertsson 2006). According to a study, the annual number of revisions of knee-joint prostheses in the USA will double from 2005 to 2015 and the number of revisions of hip-joint prostheses will double by 2026. By 2030 the frequency of knee and hip joint revisions should increase by 601% to 268,200 operations or by 137% to 96,700 operations respectively compared with 2005 (Kurtz et al. 2006). The expected massive rise of the demand for revision arthroplasties represents a major medical, health-economic and technological challenge.

The most important reason for revision is loosening of the prosthesis, with aseptic loosening at about 75% being ahead of septic loosening as the reason for revision of the hip joint (Kärrholm et al. 2007). The incidence of revisions due to periprosthetic infections is increasing. Improved surgical techniques, the introduction of bone cements containing antibiotics in the 1970s and advanced hygiene have reduced infection rates for primary joint replacements from 5–10% in the 1960s to less than 1% (Blom et al. 2003; Soderman et al. 2000). Optimized diagnostic methods allow earlier detection of periprosthetic infections, which means that prosthetic loosening is more frequently classified as septic than in the past (Tunney et al. 1999). Careful and speedy sampling and packaging, rapid transport and a long culturing time (Neut et al. 2003) are preconditions for an exact identification of possibly existing bacteria. Detaching the biofilm by means of ultrasound, the use of immunofluorescence microscopy and PCR (detection of bacterial 16S-rRNA) as well as the intraoperative frozen section technology (Tunney et al. 1999; Musso et al. 2003) are numbered among the supplementary diagnostic methods. Pathogen determination and selection of the antibiotic treatment already before the operation are expedient (Frommelt 2004).

Microbes from human skin flora are the most common cause of infections. Gram-positive bacteria in particular have a high affinity to foreign surfaces. They include staphylococci (42–66%) and streptococci (9–10%) (Zimmerli et al. 2004; Frommelt and Kühn 2005). Gram-negative bacteria such as E. coli or Pseudomonas are responsible for up to 6% of the infections of prostheses. Infections with anaerobes are acquiring increasing significance.

Revision operations represent a challenge for surgeons since they involve a higher risk of complications in comparison to the first implantation. An increased risk of infection of around 5–8% stands in the foreground in this case. This generally increased postoperative rate of infections can be reduced by the use of bone cement containing antibiotics (Frommelt 2004; Zimmerli et al. 2004; Parvizi et al. 2008). One clinically well-proven example is the COPAL® G+C revision cement (Heraeus Medical, Wehrheim). COPAL® C+C contains gentamicin and clindamycin, two antibiotics that have a synergistic bactericidal effect on more than 90% of all bacteria that can be encountered in infections in joint surgery (Frommelt and Kühn 2005; Kühn 2000). Locally antimicrobial COPAL® G+C is used for fixation of prosthetic components in revision of prostheses for prosthetic loosening and is the bone cement of choice especially in previously infected prostheses (Frommelt and Kühn 2005; Gehrke et al. 2001). In addition, this cement is used for producing bone-cement spacers for the purpose of suppressing infection in two-stage revision operations. COPAL® G+C also offers protection against infection in the course of alloarthroplastic first operations, e.g. in immune-suppressed patients.

The pharmacokinetic properties of COPAL® G+C have been thoroughly investigated in a study (Frommelt and Kühn 2005; Gehrke et al. 2001). The present observational study had the objective of documenting experience with the use of COPAL® G+C in clinical practice under everyday conditions. The investigation demonstrates the spectrum of application of an industrially produced revision cement containing antibiotics and provides information about the surgical procedure for revision operations based on actual case studies. The investigation is also intended to provide some information on how effective the revision cement is when used in revision arthroplasty.

Methods

A total of 27 patients of 15 participating physicians from 15 different hospitals and departments of surgery, emergency surgery, orthopaedics, arthroplasty or surgical rheumatology in Germany (n = 8), Austria (n = 2), the Czech Republic (n = 2) and Spain (n = 3) were included in the observational study. The physicians reported about the preoperative situation, the revision surgery and postoperative development based on a questionnaire. The patients were included on decision of the participating physicians in terms of single or two-stage revision surgery. For treatment the COPAL® bone cement containing two antibiotics was used. 40 g COPAL® contain 1 g gentamicin as gentamicin sulphate and 1 g clindamycin as clindamycin hydrochloride.

Twelve of the 27 patients were women, 15 were men. On average (± SD) the patients were 66.3 ± 12.1 years old (range 26–79). The average body weight was (± SD) 82.5 ± 17.9 kg (range 53–133), the average height (± SD) was 168.6 ± 9.8 cm (range 146–182). ◘ Table 10.1 shows the diagnoses that had led to first total joint replacement. In 14

◘ **Table 10.1.** Diagnoses before first joint replacement

Localization	Diagnosis	n
Knee	Primary gonarthrosis	9
	Posttraumatic gonarthrosis	4
	Bechterew's disease	1
	No information	5
	Total	19
Hip	Primary coxarthrosis	6
	Groin abscess/empyema	1
	Ewing sarcoma	1
	Total	8

patients the right joint was affected, in 13 patients the left joint. For 26 patients it was a single or two-stage revision, in one case it was the first implantation of a prosthesis in an infected knee joint.

The data of the report on application were subjected to a descriptive analysis.

Results

Reasons for Revision

The most frequent reason for revision surgery was an infection, with a total of 23 joints or prostheses being infected at the time of the first operation (◘ Table 10.2). There was an infection in 15 of the 19 knee prostheses, in 4 loosening without infection and in 3 patients there was both loosening of the prosthesis and infection. 1 patient suffered from suppurative arthritis of the knee joint. All 8 patients with hip implants had an infection, 4 patients were included in the report with an infection-suppressed Girdlestone situation. One patient had a fistulated infection of a femoral implant. 8 patients (38%) previously had revision surgeries or replacement of the prosthesis (hip 5 patients, knee 3 patients).

The most common accompanying diseases were arterial hypertension in 10 patients, obesity in 4 patients and type-2 diabetes in 3 patients.

and in some cases at rest while 19 patients had in part significantly reduced mobility. Eight patients with knee implants had an effusion when physically examined, 12 patients with knee- and hip-joint replacement as well as the patient with fistulating prosthetic infection had local signs of infection such as reddening or overheating. One patient had fever.

The technical examinations with imaging procedures did not give a clear indication of infection as a rule, the diagnoses were frequently not in agreement with the laboratory examinations and the microbiological results. In particular, preoperative routine X-rays did not indicate infection in half of the 23 infected prostheses and joints. In 3 out of 4 documented leucocyte scintigraphies there were indications of an infection in the region of the affected joint. In contrast to this, the laboratory results for 14 patients before the first operation clearly indicated an infection (no information for 10 patients) with increased values of the C-reactive protein (CRP) and 3 patients also had leucocytosis. Microbiologically preoperative evidence of bacteria was available from prior operations or biopsy specimens in 14 patients.

The laboratory chemical inflammation parameters were in the normal range before the second surgery in patients who were operated on in two stages.

Preoperative Symptoms and Diagnoses

The current symptoms had started between 2 months and 5 years previously, on average 18 months. 19 patients reported pain under load

Revision Operation

The revision surgeries were conducted in two stages in 20 cases and in one stage in 7 cases. The first implantation in the case of suppurative

◘ **Table 10.2.** Diagnoses for the surgery

Diagnosis	ICD-10	Localization	n
Mechanical complication due to prosthesis (loosening)	T84.0	Knee	4
		Hip	0
Infection and inflammatory reaction due to the prosthesis	T84.5	Knee	15
		Hip	8
Suppurative arthritis	M00.9	Knee	1
		Hip	0

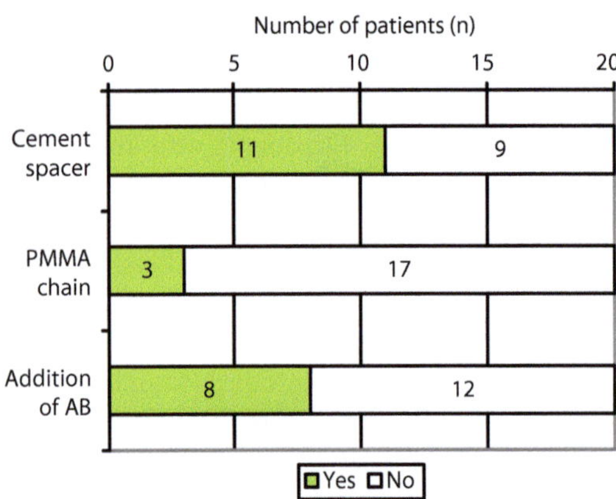

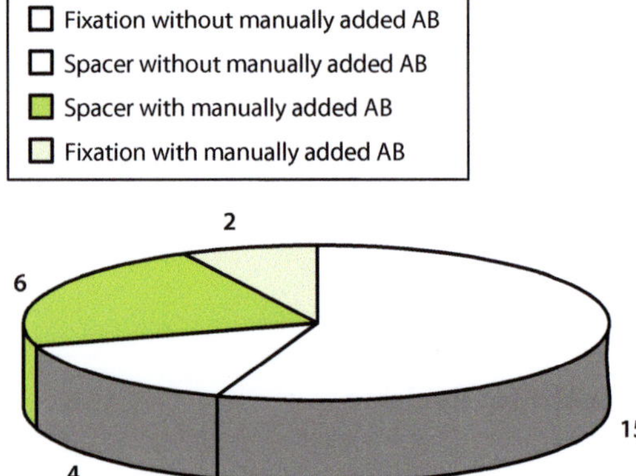

Fig. 10.1. Details of the surgical procedure in patients with two-stage revision surgeries (n = 20)

Fig. 10.2. Frequency of the addition of further antibiotics to the COPAL® bone cement used (n = 27). *AB* antibiotic

arthritis was also a one-stage revision. Bone cement spacers were inserted a total of 11 times (Fig. 10.1). Nine of the bone-cement spacers were inserted as temporary replacement in the knee joint, 2 in the hip. Two patients were treated for the interim period with a knee-joint-application prosthesis. Three patients with infected hip prostheses received temporary gentamicin PMMA chains for local antimicrobial therapy. A Girdlestone situation was created in 4 patients in the course of the disease.

All patients received either prostheses that were cemented with use of the revision cement, or spacers that were produced from this. Additional antibiotics were mixed into the bone cement for 8 patients (Fig. 10.1), and in 6 of the 8 cases spacers were produced from this mixture. The following antibiotics were added: In 4 cases vancomycin, in 1 case vancomycin and gentamicin, in 1 case vancomycin and clindamycin (Fig. 10.2). For the 2 patients without use of a spacer, vancomycin was added to the bone cement that was used for fixing the prosthesis. 4 patients received a bone cement spacer without addition of further antibiotics. Antibiotics were added manually according to published standard procedures (Frommelt 2007; Kühn 2007).

The surgeons used on average 68 g bone cement for anchoring the prostheses in the region of the knee joints (range 40–200 g), on average 71 g (range 40–120 g) in the region of the hip joints. Knee-joint spacers were formed on average from 140 g bone cement (range 60–200 g). One of the two hip joint spacers was made from 160 g bone cement, the information for the second is not available.

Germs could be detected on biopsies taken from 6 patients during the surgery. No bacteria could be detected before the operation in 4 of these patients, for 6 patients with confirmed presence of bacteria before the operation the cultures in the surgical smear preparation were sterile, and in 2 patients different bacteria were detected from those found in the preoperative biopsies. Table 10.3 shows which bacteria were present before surgery and in smears taken during the operation. More than one type of bacterium was detected in 5 patients. No information or inadequate information on the type and conduct of the smears and the duration of culturing is available.

The participating physicians preferred a commercially available vacuum mixing system as mixing method: The bone cement was mixed in 17 patients (63%) in vacuum, in 10 patients (37%) manually (hips: 4 in vacuum, 4 manually mixed; knee: 13 in vacuum, 6 manually mixed). Jet lavage was used for thorough removal of bone, blood and tissue particles in more than 80% of the patients.

Table 10.3. Preoperatively (smear or biopsy) and intraoperatively (smear) detected bacteria according to frequency

Bacterium	Sensitive to*			Number of patients with the bacterium (n)	
	Gentamicin	Clindamycin	Vancomycin	Preoperatively	Intraoperatively
Staphylococcus epidermidis	+	+	+	4	1
Staphylococcus aureus	+	+	+	4	1
Beta-hemolysin streptococci (groups B or G)	–	+	+	3	1
Enterococcus faecalis	+	–	+/–	2	2
Propionibacterium acnes	+	+	+	2	0
Coagulase-negative staphylococci	+	+	+	2	0
Dermabacter hominis	+/–	+/–	+	1	0
Streptococci of the viridans group	–	+	+	1	0
Staphylococcus chromogenes	+	+	+	1	0
Streptococci (without information on species)	–	+	+	1	0
Streptococcus parasanguinis	–	+	+	0	1
Streptococcus salivarius	–	+	+	0	1
Pseudomonas aeruginosa	+	+	–	0	1
Candida albicans	–	–	–	0	1

+ sensitive; – not sensitive; +/– limited sensitivity. *Frommelt and Kühn 2005; Gehrke 1998.

Postoperative Situation

At the time of discharge 19 patients had no pain at the wound, and delayed healing was reported in 2 patients. Clinical signs of infection were not found in 20 patients postoperatively. An infection with Pseudomonas aeruginosa, Enterococcus faecalis and Candida albicans persisted in 1 patient after implantation of a spacer, so that several spacer changes were still required in the further course of treatment (no information for 6 patients). Effusion was reported in 2 patients with knee-joint revision.

Radiological results showed normal position of the joint prosthesis or the spacer in all patients. There were no obvious indications of continuing infectious conditions. Laboratory tests showed no signs of infection processes after revision surgery, except for one patient. CRP and leucocytes were normal in 14 patients (52%), one or both inflammation parameters were increased in 2 patients and still high but clearly reducing in 8 patients (47%) (no information for 2 patients).

Conduction of systemic antibiotic treatment and/or prophylaxis was documented in a total of 13 patients, 11 of whom were operated on in two stages and 2 in a single stage. Out of the patients with two-stage revisions 10 patients received antibiotic therapy (7 patients during the interim phase, 4 patients after (re)implantation of the prosthesis), and 4 patients received prophylaxis. Out of the patients with single-stage revision surgery 1 patient received postoperative antibiotic therapy and 1 patient antibiotic prophylaxis. 14 patients were without information on antibiotic treatment or did not receive systemic antibiotic treatment (Fig. 10.3).

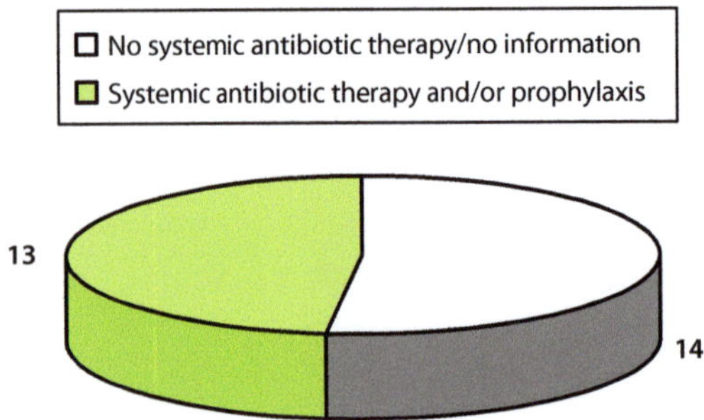

Fig. 10.3. Proportion of patients with systemic antibiotic therapy and prophylaxis (n = 27)

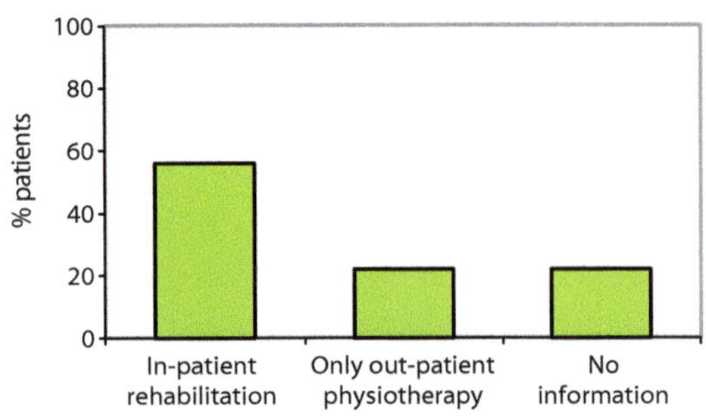

Fig. 10.4. Number of patients with in-patient or out-patient rehabilitation

Table 10.4. Duration of antibiotic therapy and prophylaxis

Antibiotics	Duration
Antibiotic treatment	
Clindamycin oral	6 days
Lincomycin i.v.	10 days
Penicillin G oral	2 weeks
Vancomycin and rifampicin i.v.	2 weeks
Penicillin G oral, followed by loracarbef oral	4 (2 + 2) weeks
Amoxicillin/clavulanic acid i.v.	5 weeks
Prophylaxis	
Ciprofloxacin oral	8 weeks
Benzathin penicillin i.m.	12 months, 6 months

The duration of antibiotic therapy was 6 days to 5 weeks; the duration of additional antibiotic long-term prophylaxis in 4 patients was between 8 weeks and 1 year (Table 10.4). For therapy the following antibiotics were used: combination of vancomycin and rifampicin i.v., combination of levofloxacin and rifampicin, lincomycin, penicillin G i.v., amoxicillin/clavulanic acid i.v., combination of cloxacillin and gentamicin, loracarbef oral, or clindamycin oral. For long-term prophylaxis benzathin penicillin i.m. or ciprofloxacin oral were used.

Rehabilitation and Result of Revision

The participating physicians reported a good result without complications around 2–10 months after the revision for 16 patients. There were no signs of infection or only moderate local problems. The patients could climb stairs for several floors or walk 1,000 meters on the roller or with walking aids. In 4 cases the physicians reported difficulty with mobilization and problems during rehabilitation, such as repeated swelling and temporary heating of the joint (no information for 7 patients). 15 patients were referred as a rule for 3 weeks for in-patient rehabilitation, which was followed partially by out-patient physiotherapy (Fig. 10.4). In-patient rehabilitation was conducted primarily for patients from Germany, for 6 patients exclusively out-patient rehabilitation that consisted primarily of physiotherapy.

Mobilization was regular for 18 patients, difficult mobilization or severe immobility was reported for 3 patients (no information for 6 patients).

Discussion

The results of the present observational study reflect the current clinical procedure for revision arthroplasty. They emphasize the relevance of infection as the cause of complications in arthroplasty and the significance of bone cement with antibiotics for treatment and prophylaxis of infections in revision arthroplasty.

The diagnosis of periprosthetic infections remains a challenge. Although some signs of infection may be detected, e.g., by imaging procedures, no single diagnostic modality alone is able to confirm infection with absolute sensitivity and specificity. Accurate diagnosis therefore often requires the use of combination of different tests and a strong clinical suspicion (Bauer et al. 2006).

The main approaches for the diagnosis of periprosthetic infection are (Bauer et al. 2006):

- symptoms and signs, e.g., joint pain,
- serologic tests, e.g., white blood-cell count, CRP,
- imaging, e.g., X-ray, labelled white blood-cell scan,
- aspiration and culture of joint fluid.

The determination of parameters of infection and inflammation in the laboratory, particularly CRP, appears to be more promising (Sanzen and Carlsson 1989; White et al. 1998; Spangehl et al. 1999). However, most serologic tests are difficult to interpret when the patient has an underlying inflammatory arthropathy (Bauer et al. 2006). As shown in the results of this observational study, increased CRP values indicate current infectious processes, such as prosthetic infection. Microbiological examination of biopsy specimens is of great importance for successful and targeted treatment of periprosthetic infections (Neut et al. 2003). Identification of bacteria is also decisive for further therapy planning – apart from the general situation of the patient. In the present study there was positive detection of bacteria preoperatively in more than half of the patients. The microbial spectrum of prosthetic infections corresponded here essentially to the spectrum known from the literature (Trampuz and Zimmerli 2005). Microbes of the human skin flora are typical of those that reach the implant during surgery. Frequent bacteria include streptococci and staphylococci. While in most cases there was polymicrobial infection of the prosthesis (Neut et al. 2003), only two patients in this study had two or more types of bacteria. No conclusions could be drawn in this study about the possible influence of transport and culture conditions on the sensitivity of the bacterial detection process.

The use of prophylactic antibiotics, laminar airflow, and other precautions have helped to reduce the incidence of clinically detected periprosthetic infection to less than 1% in a number of series (Fitzgerald 1992; Peersman et al. 2001). Addition of antibiotics to PMMA cement with demonstrable elution over a period of time has been shown to be very effective in the treatment of established periprosthetic infections (Josefsson and Kolmert 1993; Espehaug et al. 1997; Jamsen et al. 2009; Sheng et al. 2006). Accordingly, the meta-analysis of Parvizi et al. (2008) demonstrated a clear benefit especially of antibiotic cement preparations in primary total hip arthroplasty, with a significant 50% reduction in the infection rate following primary hip arthroplasty. In addition, the incidence of revision surgery was lower when using antibiotic-loaded cement. Furthermore, also in one-step exchange or two-stage revisions of infected hip implants, cements loaded with antibiotic combinations or targeted antibiotics lowered infections rates by approx. 40% (Parvizi et al. 2008).

While aseptic implant loosening is normally the primary reason for revision procedures (Kärrholm et al. 2007), the present study included primarily patients with known infections. Only 4 patients had primary aseptic implant loosening without indication of infection. It must be assumed that a selection bias was operating here and that patients who would benefit from use of a revision cement containing two antibiotics had preference in the selection process. However, it is now known that periprosthetic infections can be detected better with optimized diagnostics. This means that more cases of prosthetic loosening which previously were still classified as »aseptic« are in fact due to unrecognized occult infections and will be diagnosed in the future as septic (Tunney et al. 1999).

The postoperative period and rehabilitation and postoperative care were without complications for the majority of patients and there were no signs of renewed infection. This finding confirms that the infection rate of revision surgeries in arthroplasty can be reduced by the use of bone cement containing antibiotics (Frommelt and Kühn 2005; Kühn 2007; Buchholz and Engelbrecht 1970). Antibiotics such as gentamicin and clindamycin mixed in the revision cement are confirmed to prevent colonization of the prosthesis material by pathogenic organisms, the formation of a biofilm and therefore periprosthetic infection (van de Belt

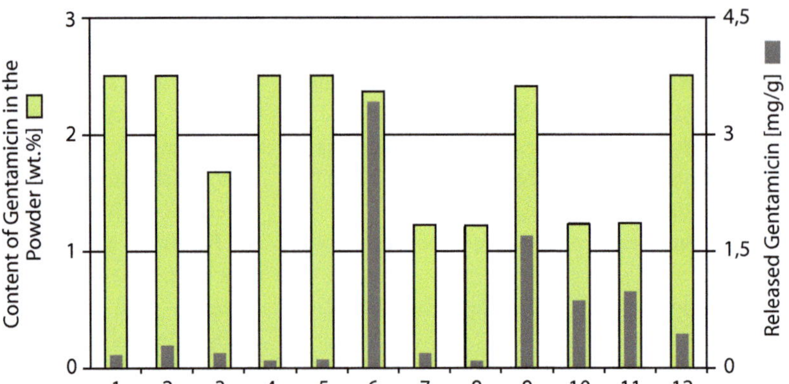

Fig. 10.5. Accumulated release of gentamicin within 7 days from different commercially available bone cements. (1–12; Modified from Kühn et al. 2005)

et al. 2001; Gristina et al. 1991). Although the bone cements that are currently available commercially have the same chemical basis, acrylic bone cements are not all alike. In the case antibiotic-loaded bone cements, e.g., elution of antimicrobial agents depends on the sort of bone cement, the properties of the antibiotics and the method of preparing the cement (Frommelt and Kühn 2005). The high-viscosity PMMA bone cement COPAL® G+C used in this study is characterized by a high content of gentamicin and clindamycin. Moreover, COPAL® G+C exhibits a very high release of antibiotics (Kühn 2007; Kühn et al. 2005; Fig. 10.5), which is a prerequisite for high local antimicrobial efficacy particularly in revision surgery.

The addition of further locally effective antibiotics appears to be justified only in exceptional cases as indicated by the microbial results. The question of the extent to which patients benefit from systemic antibiotic therapy or prophylaxis remains open. While the data of the Norwegian Arthroplasty Register indicate that supplementary systemic antibiotic administration results in the lowest revision rate (Engesaeter et al. 2003), in this study only 11 patients received such systemic antibiotic treatment.

The surgeries in most patients were conducted in two stages, which conforms to the current standard (Garvin and Hanssen 1995; Elson 1993). In almost one half of all cases a spacer was placed as a temporary solution for the interim period, 4 patients were left in the Girdlestone situation with

infection suppressed until re-implantation of the prosthesis. Implantation of a spacer made of bone cement containing antibiotics is a useful strategy for surgical management of infected implants. This procedure eliminates microbes in the region of the infected prosthesis and at the same time retains joint function. This increases the chances of long-term success of the second procedure. As the example of one patient shows, a good result can be achieved even after several years of spacer insertion. PMMA chains containing antibiotics represent in two-stage revisions an effective alternative to the use of spacer prostheses with added antibiotics. The participating physicians preferred vacuum mixing as the mixing procedure for the bone cement to obtain homogeneously mixed bone cement. Jet lavage for cleaning the bone bed was a standard part of the procedure and was used in 81% of the revision surgeries.

Infections that are associated with surgical implants such as orthopaedic devices have significant clinical and economic consequences and often result in serious disabilities (Darouiche 2004). In particular, periprosthetic infection is associated with an immense physiological and psychological cost for the patient and a high financial burden for healthcare systems (Zimmerli et al. 2004; Parvizi et al. 2008; Bauer et al. 2006). In a study, the average cost of combined medical and surgical treatment for one arthroplasty infection has been estimated to $ 30,000 in the U.S. (Darouiche 2004). The use of antibiotic-loaded bone cements, which has been shown to lower infection rates by 40–50% (Parvizi et al. 2008), may result in a considerable reduction of overall cost of treating implant-associated infections.

The results of this observational study indicate that the application of a revision cement containing antibiotics in revision arthroplasty is associated with a favourable outcome. Both infected knee and hip total prostheses with protracted problems in some cases can be improved with various procedures, including local and systemic administration of antibiotics.

Literature

Bauer TW, Parvizi J, Kobayashi N, Krebs V (2006) Diagnosis of periprosthetic infection. J Bone Joint Surg Am 88: 869-882

Blom AW, Taylor AH, Pattison G, Whitehouse S, Bannister GC (2003) Infection after total hip arthroplasty. The Avon experience. J Bone Joint Surg Br 85: 956-959

Buchholz H, Engelbrecht H (1970) Über die Depotwirkung einiger Antibiotika bei Vermischung mit dem Kunstharz Palacos. Chirurg 41: 511-515

Bundesgeschäftsstelle Qualitätssicherung GGmbH (2006) Hüft-Endoprothesen-Erstimplantation. http://www.bqs-outcome.de/2006/ergebnisse/leistungsbereiche/hueft_endo_erst/download

Bundesgeschäftsstelle Qualitätssicherung GGMBH (2007) Knie-Totalendoprothesen-Erstimplantation. http://www.bqs-outcome.de/2007/ergebnisse/leistungsbereiche/knie_tep_erst/index_html

Darouiche RO (2004) Treatment of infections associated with surgical implants. N Engl J Med 350: 1422-1429

Elson RA (1993) Exchange arthroplasty for infection. Perspectives from the United Kingdom. Orthop Clin North Am 24: 761-767

Engesaeter LB, Lie SA, Espehaug B, Furnes O, Vollset SE, Havelin LI (2003) Antibiotic prophylaxis in total hip arthroplasty: effects of antibiotic prophylaxis systemically and in bone cement on the revision rate of 22,170 primary hip replacements followed 0-14 years in the Norwegian Arthroplasty Register. Acta Orthop Scand 74: 644-651

Espehaug B, Engesaeter LB, Vollset SE, Havelin LI, Langeland N (1997) Antibiotic prophylaxis in total hip arthroplasty. Review of 10,905 primary cemented total hip replacements reported to the Norwegian arthroplasty register, 1987 to 1995. J Bone Joint Surg Br 79: 590-595

Fitzgerald RH Jr (1992) Total hip arthroplasty sepsis. Prevention and diagnosis. Orthop Clin North Am 23: 259-264

Frommelt L (2004) Lokale Antibiotikatherapie. In: Schnettler S (Hrsg) Septische Knochenchirurgie. Thieme, Stuttgart, New York, S 82-90

Frommelt L (2007) Antibiotic choices in bone surgery - local therapy using antibiotic-loaded bone cement. In: Walenkamp GHIM (ed) Local antibiotics in arthroplasty. State of the art from an interdisciplinary view. Thieme, Stuttgart New York, pp 59-64

Frommelt L, Kühn KD (2005) Antibiotic-loaded cement. In: Breusch SJ, Malchau M (eds) The well-cemented total hip arthroplasty. Springer, Berlin Heidelberg New York Tokyo, pp 86-92

Garvin KL, Hanssen AD (1995) Infection after total hip arthroplasty. Past, present, and future. J Bone Joint Surg Am 77: 1576-1588

Gehrke T (1998) Neuer antibiotikahaltiger Knochenzement. Medizin Forum aktuell 64

Gehrke T, v. Foerster G, Frommelt L, Marx A (2001) Pharmacokinetic study of a gentamicin/clindamycin bone cement used in one-stage revision arthroplasty. In: Walenkamp GHIM, Murray DW (eds) Bone cements and cementing technique. Springer, Berlin Heidelberg New York Tokyo, pp 127-134

Gristina AG, Naylor PT, Myrvik QN (1991) Mechanisms of musculoskeletal sepsis. Orthop Clin North Am 22: 363-371

Jamsen E, Huhtala H, Puolakka T, Moilanen T (2009) Risk factors for infection after knee arthroplasty. A register-based analysis of 43,149 cases. J Bone Joint Surg Am 91: 38-47

Josefsson G, Kolmert L (1993) Prophylaxis with systematic antibiotics versus gentamicin bone cement in total hip arthroplasty. A ten-year survey of 1,688 hips. Clin Orthop Relat Res 210-214

Kärrholm J, Garellick G, Rogmark C, Herberts P (2007) The Swedish hip arthroplasty register. Annual Report 2006. [Internet] http://www.jru.orthop.gu.se/2007

Kühn KD (2000) Bone cements. Up-to-date comparison of physical and chemical properties of commercial materials. Springer, Berlin, Heidelberg New York Tokyo

Kühn KD (2007) Antibiotic-loaded bone cements – antibiotic release and influence on mechanical properties. In: Walenkamp GHIM, ed. Local antibiotics in arthroplasty. State of the art from an interdisciplinary view. Thieme, Stuttgart, New York, pp 47-58

Kühn KD, Ege W, Gopp U (2005) Acrylic bone cements: composition and properties. Orthop Clin North Am 36: 17-28

Kurtz S, Lau E, Zhao K, Mowat F, Ong K, Halpern M (2006) The future burden of hip and knee revisions. US projections from 2005 to 2030. 73rd Meeting of the American Academy of Orthopaedic Surgeons. Chicago, USA

Lidgren L, Robertsson O (2006) The Swedish Knee Arthroplasty Register 2005. Department of Orthopedics, Lund University Hospital

Musso AD, Mohanty K, Spencer-Jones R (2003) Role of frozen section histology in diagnosis of infection during revision arthroplasty. Postgrad Med J 79: 590-593

Neut D, van Horn JR, van Kooten TG, van der Mei HC, Busscher HJ (2003) Detection of biomaterial-associated infections in orthopaedic joint implants. Clin Orthop Relat Res 261-268

Parvizi J, Saleh KJ, Ragland PS, Pour AE, Mont MA (2008) Efficacy of antibiotic-impregnated cement in total hip replacement. Acta Orthop 79: 335-341

Peersman G, Laskin R, Davis J, Peterson M (2001) Infection in total knee replacement: a retrospective review of 6489 total knee replacements. Clin Orthop Relat Res 15-23

Sanzen L, Carlsson AS (1989) The diagnostic value of C-reactive protein in infected total hip arthroplasties. J Bone Joint Surg Br 71: 638-641

Sculco TP (1993) The economic impact of infected total joint arthroplasty. Instr Course Lect 42: 349-351

Sheng PY, Konttinen L, Lehto M et al. (2006) Revision total knee arthroplasty: 1990 through 2002. A review of the Finnish arthroplasty registry. J Bone Joint Surg Am 88: 1425-1430

Soderman P, Malchau H, Herberts P (2000) Outcome after total hip arthroplasty: Part I. General health evaluation in relation to definition of failure in the Swedish National Total Hip Arthoplasty register. Acta Orthop Scand 71: 354-359

Spangehl MJ, Masri BA, O'Connell JX, Duncan CP (1999) Prospective analysis of preoperative and intraoperative investigations for the diagnosis of infection at the sites of two hundred and two revision total hip arthroplasties. J Bone Joint Surg Am 81: 672-683

The Institute for Orthopaedics (2008) The 2007-2008 orthopaedics industry annual report. Chagrin Falls, Ohio, USA

Trampuz A, Zimmerli W (2005) Prosthetic joint infections: update in diagnosis and treatment. Swiss Med Wkly 135: 243-251

Tunney MM, Patrick S, Curran MD, et al. (1999) Detection of prosthetic hip infection at revision arthroplasty by immunofluorescence microscopy and PCR amplification of the bacterial 16S rRNA gene. J Clin Microbiol 37: 3281-3290

van de Belt H, Neut D, Schenk W, van Horn JR, van der Mei HC, Busscher HJ (2001) Infection of orthopedic implants and the use of antibiotic-loaded bone cements. A review. Acta Orthop Scand 72: 557-571

White J, Kelly M, Dunsmuir R (1998) C-reactive protein level after total hip and total knee replacement. J Bone Joint Surg Br 80: 909-911

Zimmerli W, Trampuz A, Ochsner PE (2004) Prosthetic-joint infections. N Engl J Med 351: 1645-1654

Treatment of an Infected Joint Prosthesis: Difficult Challenge for an Orthopedist Surgeon

Thomas Bauer, Alain Lortat-Jacob

To manage an infected arthroplasty remains a challenge for the physician both for the diagnosis and for the treatment. For the infectious disease physician, the main problem is to assess with accuracy the present infection according to the history of the patient, to clinical and biological data, and to look for distant infectious foci. Moreover, he has to control the efficacy and tolerance of the antibiotic therapy. For the microbiologist, the challenge is to identify with accuracy the infecting agents and to make the difference within contamination and real infection. For the anesthesiologist, the problem is to analyze the general conditions of the patient before surgery in order to know which type of surgery and anesthesia would be optimal for the patient. For the orthopedist surgeon, the difficulty is not only to know if the implant has to be removed in a one or two-stage protocol, but the challenge is to be able to have a perfect cleaning of bone and soft tissues in order to control the infection and to make a perfect reconstruction in order to achieve good functional results. He has to adapt to each patient with local and general differences. In these conditions, the management of an infected joint implant imposes a multidisciplinary staff.

The first difficulty when dealing with septic arthroplasties is for the diagnosis. For most of the cases, the situation is clear with clinical, radiographic, biological and microbiological findings making the diagnosis of infection certain. However in some cases all the data cannot be gathered together and the diagnosis of infection is more uncertain. The best example is the low-grade infection without evident clinical or biological symptoms and with only microbiological findings on intraoperative samples; for this situation it is sometimes unclear if the diagnosis is a mechanical failure of the prosthesis with contamination of deep samples or a real deep infection of the prosthesis. Another very disturbing situation for the physician is the case of an infected implant without microbiological findings and negative cultures. For these unclear situations, new microbiological techniques can perhaps help the physician for the diagnosis. Unfortunately, often new sophisticated techniques (PCR, ultrasonication etc.) do not allow to strictly conclude on the question whether the implant is infected or not and increase the preoperative doubt. In order to avoid these unclear situations for the diagnosis, all the pre- and intraoperative deep samples must be taken after a long delay without any antibiotics. Antibiotics alone without surgery may lead to an increased difficulty to establish the diagnosis of infection.

Another difficulty remains with the choice of the optimal surgical and medical treatment for each patient. Regarding the microorganisms infecting the implants, the question is not only on the bacterial resistance against antibiotics but on mechanical properties (with adherence to implants) and diagnosis of deep sepsis foci spreading to the implants too. Thus, antibiotic therapy for the treatment of an infected joint implant is very difficult in its choice, adaptation, level, survey and length. It depends on the sensitivity of the microorganisms, on local, general conditions and on the history of the infection (acute, chronic, recurrence, surgical procedure). The antibiogram is only a small part of the identification of the microorganism infecting a joint prosthesis and does not give information on the history of the infection and therapeutic options already attempted.

During surgery, the difficulty is to be sure to have a perfect cleaning of all the bony surfaces and soft tissues. It often imposes large approaches with osteotomies (femorotomy, trochanterotomy, osteotomy of the anterior tibial tuberosity) and increases the risk of mechanical problems after reconstruction. Debridement, synovectomy and bone excision are difficult and the quality of the cleaning is linked to the experience of the surgeon in bone and joint infections.

Microbiological staffs with microbiologists, infectious disease physicians, anesthesiologists and orthopedist surgeons must be the gold standard for all the discussions about diagnosis and therapeutic options when dealing with a septic arthroplasty. These staffs enable to consider the overall patients' problems and not only a microbiological problem or a bone reconstruction difficulty.

The latest difficulty with infections on joint prostheses is to know when the infection can be considered as healed. With a long follow-up among cohorts of patients treated for sepsis on arthroplasties, septic recurrences appear, with same microorganisms or with different strains. Precise criteria of healing are lacking for infection on arthroplasty.

Low-Grade Infection and Multiresistant Gram-Positive Cocci

Reiner Schaumann, Arne C. Rodloff

Introduction

Loosening of the prosthetic joint replacement due to aseptic mechanic failures and late infections are the most common problems and limiting factors after total joint prostheses. The infections are often low-grade without unequivocal systemic signs and symptoms of an infection caused by less virulent bacteria. Despite good microbiological culture standards, the detection of the bacteria is often a challenge. Moreover, other invasive and non-invasive diagnostic procedures also fail in diagnosing low-grade infections. However, the discrimination between septic and aseptic loosening confirmed by microbiological findings is important for an adequate treatment. Coagulase-negative staphylococci, especially multiresistant *Staphylococcus epidermidis* (MRSE), are the most common isolated bacteria in the infected patients. Other resistant gram-positive cocci isolated are vancomycin-resistant enterococci (VRE) and the more virulent methicillin-resistant *S. aureus* (MRSA). In addition to surgical intervention, treatment of the infections needs local and systemic administration of appropriate antimicrobial agents that are capable of achieving sufficient drug concentration at the site of infection.

Diagnosis of Low-Grade Infections

Periprosthetic infection is a rare but serious complication after prosthetic joint replacement (Frommelt 2006; Zimmerli and Ochsner 2003). The infection rate is estimated to be 0.5 to 2% (Zimmerli and Ochsner 2003; Laffer et al. 2006; Zimmerli et al. 2004). On the other hand, loosening of the prosthetic joint replacement due to aseptic mechanic failures and late infections are the most common problems and limiting factors after total joint prostheses (Ince et al. 2004; Nilsdotter-Augustinsson et al. 2007). Furthermore, the discrimination between septic and aseptic loosening is important for an adequate treatment since in septic loosening the surgical therapy needs to be supported by the administration of antimicrobial agents (Ince et al. 2004). For appropriate antimicrobial treatment, isolation, identification, and susceptibility testing of the pathogenic microorganism is necessary (Schäfer et al. 2008). According to an accepted classification, early infections occur within the first 4 weeks after implantation of a joint replacement (Schäfer et al. 2008). In contrast to late infections, these infections are often caused by more virulent microorganisms such as *S. aureus* causing local and systemic signs and symptoms of an infection (Schäfer et al. 2008). However; in a retrospective analysis of 90 patients with total knee replacement all of them developed postoperatively pyrexia and sixteen patients developed a temperature higher than 39 °C. None of the 16 patients had evidence of infection (Kennedy et al. 1997). Late infections after total joint prostheses are often low-grade without unequivocal systemic signs and symptoms of an infection and are caused by less virulent bacteria such as coagulase-negative staphylococci (Schäfer et al. 2008). The detection of these bacteria is often a challenge despite good microbiological culture standards (Ince et al. 2004; Clarke et al. 2004). However, other invasive and non-invasive diagnostic procedures such as e. g. determination of C-reactive protein, other laboratory data, and radiographs or bone scans are also often failing in diagnosing low-grade infection and are associated with both false-positive and false-negative results (Schäfer et al. 2008; Fink et al. 2008). To confirm the diagnosis prosthetic joint infection by microbiological analysis it is necessary to take multiple tissue samples (5 to 6 specimens per operation). In a study of Atkins et al. (1998), the isolation of an indistinguishable microorganism from three or more independent specimens was highly predictive of an infection (sensitivity 66%; specificity 99.6%; posttest probability of infection 96.4%). Furthermore, a recently published study has reemphasized that prolonged microbiological culture of the samples for 2 weeks is promising because it yields higher rates of positivity. »Early« detected species were mostly staphylococci and emerged predominantly during the first week, whereas »late« detected microorganisms (mostly *Probionibacterium* species) were detected mainly during the second week (Schäfer et al. 2008). PCR for detections of 16S rRNA in tissue specimens obtained from hip joints after total hip replacement seems not superior to routine bacteriologic culture technique for detection of low-grade infections (Ince et al. 2004).

Isolated Microorganisms

Microorganisms isolated from specimens of patients with prostheses joint infections are shown in ◘ Table 12.1 (Laffer et al. 2006; Frommelt 2000; Moran et al. 2007).

Emergence of Resistance

As shown in ◘ Table 12.1, in patients with prostheses infection the isolated microorganisms are in approx. 20 to 40% coagulase-negative staphylococci, in approx. 25 to 35% *S. aureus*, and in approx. 8 to 20% streptococci and enterococci, respectively. The frequency of MRSA has increased in the last years and continues to grow in hospital-associated setting as well as in community-settings and the frequency of methicillin/multiresistant coagulase-

◘ **Table 12.1.** Organisms isolated from cases of prostheses infection

Microorganism	Study		
	Laffer et al. 2006	Frommelt 2000	Moran et al. 2007
	Number of isolated microorganinsms		
	n = 40	n = 1077	n = 267
	Percent of isolates (%)		
Coagulase-negative staphylococci	22.5	41.0	30.0
S. aureus	35.0	26.2	29.6
Streptococci and enterococci	20.0	8.4	13.9
Gram-negative rods	15.0	7.4	7.5
Anaerobes including *Propionibacterium* spp.	5.0	13.7	4.9
Other	2.5	3.3	14.1

negative staphylococci especially *S. epidermidis* (MRSE) is already high (Boucher and Corey 2008; Jones et al. 2003; Rice 2006; Woodford 2005). For example, during 2001 the incidence of MRSA and MRSE causing skin and soft-tissue infections was 12.4% and 62.2% in Germany and 44.4% and 75.2% in the USA, respectively (Jones et al. 2003). The MRSA and MRSE are resistant against every β-lactam antimicrobial agent and often multiresistant. Moreover, the prevalence of vancomycin-resistant enterococci (VRE) is increasing and correlated with the consumption of vancomycin. For example, among hospitals participating in the National Nosocomial Infection Surveillance System from 1989 to 1997, the percentage of enterococci reported as resistant to vancomycin increased from 0.4% to 23.2% in intensive-care settings and from 0.3% to 15.4% in non-intensive-care settings (Martone 1998). The yearly vancomycin usage (all suppliers, all forms) rose from 7,600 kg in 1989 to 11,200 kg in 1996 in the United States (Kirst et al. 1998). The consumption of vancomycin increases due to the treatment of increasing rates of MRSA and MRSE and the treatment of antibiotic associated colitis caused by *Clostridium difficile* (AAC) with vancomycin (Kirst et al. 1998; Sakoulas and Moellering 2008).

Biofilm

The pathogenesis of prostheses infections differ from »classic« infections since the bacteria growing on an artificial surface create biofilms by building an extracellular matrix, an exopolysaccharide film. Furthermore, due to quorum-sensing signals, the bacteria switch their metabolism from planctonic growth to sessile growth. These factors protect the bacteria against antimicrobial agents and the host defence (Anderson and O'Toole 2008; von Eiff et al. 2002, 2005). Usually, susceptibility testing is performed with bacteria growing planctonically. In contrast, the minimal inhibitory concentrations (MICs) of bacteria growing in biofilm (sessile growth) against antimicrobial agents are up to 1000-fold higher compared to MICs of bacteria growing planctonically (Nishimura et al. 2006). Thus, as demonstrated for rifampicin which

penetrated biofilms by *S. epidermidis* but failed to effectively kill the bacteria, the protection of the bacteria against antimicrobial agents is not only a diffusion problem due to the extracellular matrix (Zheng and Stewart 2002).

Treatment of Low-Grade Infections

The treatment of low-grade infections needs surgical intervention and in addition is supported by local and systemic administration of appropriate antimicrobials agents that are capable of achieving sufficient drug concentration at the site of infection (Frommelt 2006). For appropriate antimicrobial treatment isolation, identification and susceptibility testing of the pathogenic microorganism is mandatory (Schäfer et al. 2008).

It is noteworthy that the concentration of antimicrobial agents in bone after systemic administration range from low to more than 100% of the serum concentration (◨ Table 12.2; Rosin et al.

◨ **Table 12.2.** Bone concentration of antimicrobial agents administered systemically compared to serum level (Rosin et al. 1974; Toma et al. 2006; Venugopalan and Martin 2007; Venugopalan et al. 2007; Wittmann 1980)

Antimicrobial agent	Approx. bone concentration compared to serum level (%)
Ampicillin	5
Methicillin	20
Cefazolin	4–18
Meropenem	93–105
Rifampicin	100
Ciprofloxacin	28–55
Clindamycin	50–100
Gentamicin	5
Fosfomycin	40
Vancomycin	14
Daptomycin	1–2 (animal model)
Linezolid	40–50
Tigecycline	35

1974; Toma et al. 2006; Venugopalan and Martin 2007; Venugopalan et al. 2007; Wittmann 1980). Thus, an appropriate level of antibiotic concentration for different antimicrobial agents is not always achievable at the site of infection.

On the other hand, locally administered antimicrobial agents (e. g. antibiotic-containing PMMA cements or beads) achieve extremely high levels of antimicrobial agents at the site of infection (Gehrke et al. 2001; Wahlig 1987; Walenkamp 1997). Walenkamp reported that the local exudates concentration after implantation of gentamicin-containing PMMA beads is much higher compared to levels achieved with gentamicin-containing spacers (Walenkamp 2007).

The release of antimicrobial agents from PMMA-cements depends on the type of cement and the formulation of the antimicrobial agent. For example, the release of gentamicin from PMMA cement ranged from less than 0.5 mg/g up to nearly 3.5 mg/g depending on the type of cement and formulation of gentamicin (Kühn 2000). Thus, it is very important to use an appropriate cement and antimicrobial agent for local treatment. Furthermore, clindamycin increase the release of gentamicin from PMMA-cements (Kühn 2000), and macrolides (and therefore probably clindamycin, too) increase the activity of vancomycin against biofilms of *S. epidermidis* due to eradication of exopolysaccharides (Peck et al. 2003). This effect is independent of the antibacterial activity of the macrolides against staphylococci (Peck et al. 2003).

Besides vancomycin, new antimicrobial agents such as linezolid, daptomycin, and tigecycline have good activity against MRSA and MRSE and the latter also against VRE (Rice 2006; Linden 2007). However, in the meantime strains resistant against linezolid, tigecycline, and daptomycin have also been described (Linden 2007; Bouchillon et al. 2008). Furthermore, vancomycin/glycopeptide intermediate and resistant *S. aureus* isolates (VISA, GISA, and VRSA, respectively) have been detected and described although the prevalence is still rare (Boucher and Corey 2008; Rice 2006; Woodford 2005; Sakoulas and Moellering 2008). Thus, the treatment of prostheses infections especially low-grade infections is getting more difficult due to the increasing incidence of resistant gram-positive microorganisms.

References

Anderson GG, O'Toole GA (2008) Innate and induced resistance mechanisms of bacterial biofilms. Curr Top Microbiol Immunol 322: 85–105

Atkins BL, Athanasou N, Deeks JJ, Crook DW, Simpson H, Peto TE, McLardy-Smith P, Berendt AR (1998) Prospective evaluation of criteria for microbiological diagnosis of prosthetic-joint infection at revision arthroplasty. The OSIRIS Collaborative Study Group. J Clin Microbiol 36: 2932–2939

Boucher HW, Corey GR (2008) Epidemiology of methicillin-resistant Staphylococcus aureus. Clin Infect Dis 46 (Suppl 5): S344–349

Bouchillon SK, Iredell JR, Barkham T, Lee K, Dowzicky MJ (2009) Comparative in vitro activity of tigecycline and other antimicrobials against Gram-negative and Gram-positive organisms collected from the Asia-Pacific Rim as part of the Tigecycline Evaluation and Surveillance Trial (TEST). Int J Antimicrob Agents 33: 130–136

Clarke MT, Lee PT, Roberts CP, Gray J, Keene GS, Rushton N (2004) Contamination of primary total hip replacements in standard and ultra-clean operating theaters detected by the polymerase chain reaction. Acta Orthop Scand 75: 544–548

Fink B, Makowiak C, Fuerst M, Berger I, Schäfer P, Frommelt L (2008) The value of synovial biopsy, joint aspiration and C-reactive protein in the diagnosis of late peri-prosthetic infection of total knee replacements. J Bone Joint Surg Br 90: 874–878

Frommelt L (2000) Periprosthetic infection – bacteria and the interface between prosthesis and bone. In: Learmonth ID (ed) Interfaces in total hip arthroplasty. Springer, London Berlin Heidelberg New York, pp 153–161

Frommelt L (2006) Principles of systemic antimicrobial therapy in foreign material associated infection in bone tissue, with special focus on periprosthetic infection. Injury 37 (Suppl 2): S87–94

Gehrke T, von Förster G, Frommelt L (2001) Pharmacokinetic study of a gentamicin/clindamycin bone cement used in one-stage revision arthroplasty. In: Walenkamp GHIM, Murray DW (eds) Bone cements and cementing technique. Springer, Berlin Heidelberg New York, pp 127–134

Ince A, Rupp J, Frommelt L, Katzer A, Gille J, Löhr JF (2004) Is »aseptic« loosening of the prosthetic cup after total hip replacement due to nonculturable bacterial pathogens in patients with low-grade infection? Clin Infect Dis 39: 1599–1603

Jones ME, Karlowsky JA, Draghi DC, Thornsberry C, Sahm DF, Nathwani D (2003) Epidemiology and antibiotic susceptibility of bacteria causing skin and soft tissue infections in the USA and Europe: a guide to appropriate antimicrobial therapy. Int J Antimicrob Agents 22: 406–419

Kennedy JG, Rodgers WB, Zurakowski D, Sullivan R, Griffin D, Beardsley W, Sheehan L (1997) Pyrexia after total knee replacement. A cause for concern? Am J Orthop 26: 549–552, 554

Kirst HA, Thompson DG, Nicas TI (1998) Historical yearly usage of vancomycin. Antimicrob Agents Chemother 42: 1303–1304

Kühn KD (2000) Bone cements. Up-to-date comparison of physical and chemical properties of commercial materials. Springer, Berlin Heidelberg New York

Laffer RR, Graber P, Ochsner PE, Zimmerli W (2006) Outcome of prosthetic knee-associated infection: evaluation of 40 consecutive episodes at a single centre. Clin Microbiol Infect 12: 433–439

Linden PK (2007) Optimizing therapy for vancomycin-resistant enterococci (VRE). Semin Respir Crit Care Med 28: 632–645

Martone WJ (1998) Spread of vancomycin-resistant enterococci: why did it happen in the United States? Infect Control Hosp Epidemiol 19: 539–545

Moran E, Masters S, Berendt AR, McLardy-Smith P, Byren I, Atkins BL (2007) Guiding empirical antibiotic therapy in orthopaedics: the microbiology of prosthetic joint infection managed by debridement, irrigation and prosthesis retention. J Infect 55: 1–7

Nilsdotter-Augustinsson Å, Briheim G, Herder A, Ljunghusen O, Wahlström O, Öhman L (2007) Inflammatory response in 85 patients with loosened hip prostheses: a prospective study comparing inflammatory markers in patients with aseptic and septic prosthetic loosening. Acta Orthop 78: 629–639

Nishimura S, Tsurumoto T, Yonekura A, Adachi K, Shindo H (2006) Antimicrobial susceptibility of Staphylococcus aureus and Staphylococcus epidermidis biofilms isolated from infected total hip arthroplasty cases. J Orthop Sci 11: 46–50

Peck KR, Kim SW, Jung SI, Kim YS, Oh WS, Lee JY, Jin JH, Kim S, Song JH, Kobayashi H (2003) Antimicrobials as potential adjunctive agents in the treatment of biofilm infection with Staphylococcus epidermidis. Chemotherapy 49: 189–193

Rice LB (2006) Antimicrobial resistance in gram-positive bacteria. Am J Infect Control 34 (Suppl 1): S11–19

Rosin H, Rosin AM, Krämer J (1974) Determination of antibiotic levels in human bone. I. Gentamicin levels in bone. Infection 2: 3–6

Sakoulas G, Moellering RC Jr (2008) Increasing antibiotic resistance among methicillin-resistant Staphylococcus aureus strains. Clin Infect Dis 46 (Suppl 5): S360–367

Schäfer P, Fink B, Sandow D, Margull A, Berger I, Frommelt L (2008) Prolonged bacterial culture to identify late periprosthetic joint infection: a promising strategy. Clin Infect Dis 47: 1403–1409

Toma MB, Smith KM, Martin CA, Rapp RP (2006) Pharmacokinetic considerations in the treatment of methicillin-resistant Staphylococcus aureus osteomyelitis. Orthopedics 29: 497–501

Venugopalan V, Martin CA (2007) Selecting anti-infective agents for the treatment of bone infections: new anti-infective agents and chronic suppressive therapy. Orthopedics 30: 832–834

Venugopalan V, Smith KM, Young MH (2007) Selecting anti-infective agents for the treatment of bone infections. Orthopedics 30: 713–717

von Eiff C, Jansen B, Kohnen W, Becker K (2005) Infections associated with medical devices: pathogenesis, management and prophylaxis. Drugs 65: 179–214

von Eiff C, Peters G, Heilmann C (2002) Pathogenesis of infections due to coagulase-negative staphylococci. Lancet Infect Dis 2: 677–685

Wahlig H (1987) Über die Freisetzung von Antibiotika aus Knochenzement – Ergebnisse vergleichender Untersuchungen in vitro und in vivo. Aktuelle Probl Chir Orthop 31: 221–226

Walenkamp GH (1997) Chronic osteomyelitis. Acta Orthop Scand 68: 497–506

Walenkamp GHIM (2007) Treatment of infected prostheses – the Dutch experience. In: Walenkamp GHIM (ed) Local antibiotics in arthroplasty. Thieme, Stuttgart New York, pp 133–143

Wittmann DH (1980) Chemotherapeutic principles of difficult-to-treat infections in surgery: II. Bone and joint infections. Infection 8: 330–333

Woodford N (2005) Biological counterstrike: antibiotic resistance mechanisms of Gram-positive cocci. Clin Microbiol Infect 11 (Suppl 3): 2–21

Zheng Z, Stewart PS (2002) Penetration of rifampin through Staphylococcus epidermidis biofilms. Antimicrob Agents Chemother 46: 900–903

Zimmerli W, Ochsner PE (2003) Management of infection associated with prosthetic joints. Infection 31: 99–108

Zimmerli W, Trampuz A, Ochsner PE (2004) Prosthetic-joint infections. N Engl J Med 351: 1645–1654

Antibiotic Strategies in Septic Arthroplasties

José Cordero-Ampuero

Introduction

Implant infections do not heal only with antibiotics: this is explained by the four mechanisms of bacterial resistance (Cordero 1999; Cordero and Garcia-Cimbrelo 2000; Cordero-Ampuero 2000):

- Implants are not vascularized, so antibodies and antibiotics do not reach adequately the infected implant and bone.
- Biomaterials reduce immune system efficiency.
- Biofilm: Bacteria adhere to implants forming resistant biofilms.
- Intracellular bacteria: Bacteria are able to survive inside different cells.

Biomaterials Reduce Immune System Efficiency

Polymethylmetacrylate (PMMA)

Although PMMA has proven clinically to be a very efficient biomaterial in primary joint arthroplasty, it reduces phagocytosis as published by Petty thirty years ago (Petty 1978). It is also the orthopaedic biomaterial more prone to infection when compared to polyethylene, stainless steel 316-SL, cobalt-chromium alloy and titanium alloy, as has been demonstrated in experimental models by the group of Petty and by us (Petty et al. 1985; Cordero and Munuera 1996).

Metals

Cytotoxic metals (as cobalt or chromium) infect with smaller bacterial inocula than biocompatible metals (as titanium and alluminum; Cordero et al. 1994).

Treatment

When considering that all biomaterials (in different degree) reduce immune-system efficiency (to a different degree), it is obvious that appropriate treatment should be the removal of all implants (including all cement). Antibiotics are not useful at all for avoiding this problem.

When considering this mechanism of bacterial resistance it is also obvious that treatment of an infected arthroplasty is better with a two-stage protocol than with a one-stage. When applying a two-stage (especially if no spacer is used) there are no remaining biomaterials inside the infected region, so microbiological healing is easier. With a one-stage protocol new biomaterials are implanted, and its pernicious effect on immune activity begins again (Cordero and Garcia-Cimbrelo 2000).

Biofilm

Biofilm Formation

Bacteria survive with a planctonic form of life (floating in a liquid media) only in some types of clinical infections. On the contrary, bacteria develop an adherent way of living when exposed to a surface, as is the case in many clinical infections (endocarditis, urethritis, prostathitis), especially when artificial implants are involved.

Bacteria, when exposed to a biomaterial, adhere to the surface. Once adhered, they begin to produce polysaccharides that are secreted outside the cell (exopolysacharides), forming a huge external cover denominated glycocalix. Glycocalix is highly hydrated and occupies a 99:1 proportion of space in respect to bacterial volume.

Bacteria multiply by mitosis under this large cover of exopolysacharides, so new layers of bacteria are formed (growing over the initial adhered), and as the process continues the biofilm is formed (Gristina et al. 1991). It is also possible that new bacteria join already-adhered bacteria: it has been demonstrated that *Pseudomonas* and *Proteus* increase adherence if *S. epidermis* are already adhered (Chang and Merritt 1994).

It has also been demonstrated that porosity (Cordero et al. 1994, 1996), as well as hydrophobicity (Donlan 2001), increase bacterial adherence.

The nutrition of bacteria living inside biofilm is different according to its longevity and position, so those in deep layers maintain a different metabolic state than those in more superficial layers.

Biofilm also allows that new and almost unknown mechanisms of intercellular communication are established. These communication processes are generically denominated as »quorum sensing«.

Demonstrating Biofilm in Orthopaedic Infection

Biofilms in orthopaedic infections were classically demonstrated by surface electron microscopy more than twenty years ago (Gristina and Costerton 1985): 76% of infected implants presented adhered bacteria. Most importantly, many of these bacteria were not identified by conventional microbiological procedures.

Very recently adherent bacteria have been demonstrated after sonication of retired implants. This is a high-sensitivity diagnostic method (Trampuz et al. 2007). Moreover, in accordance with Gristina's hypothesis, large numbers of bacteria usually non-pathogenic are adhered to implants, as demonstrated by quantitative cultures of sonicate (Esteban et al. 2008). The use of sonication, together with a broad spectrum of culture media, increases the possibilities for the diagnosis of device-related orthopaedic infections. The significance of some isolates that appeared with high colony counts, but without clinical symptoms or signs, needs further evaluation to classify them properly as contaminants or pathogens.

Biofilm as a Defensive Barrier

Biofilms inhibits immune activity by multiple mechanisms. It decreases or inhibits polymorphonuclear chemotaxis, complement activation, opsonization, phagocytosis and antibody susceptibility. All these mechanisms facilitate infection chronicity.

Treatment of Biofilms

The therapeutic strategy for adhered biofilms forces to implant removal, so adhered bacteria are taken out. In this sense, two stage as well as one stage are efficient for this mechanism of resistance.

Recently many authors consider that biofilm is formed after 24–48 hours, so it is doubtful the efficiency of »conservative surgery« (based mainly on surgical débridement) for acute infections (biofilm adhered on implants is not retired; Mihalko et al. 2008).

Antibiotics for orthopaedic infections should have a good penetration and activity against bacteria living inside biofilms.

It is long known that beta-lactam antibiotics (penicillins, cephalosporins) are not able to penetrate biofilms, so they are not useful for established infections (Arizono et al. 1992; Fischer et al. 1996).

Glycopeptides (vancomycin and teicoplanin), as are formed by chains, adhere to the exopolysaccharides of glycocalix, remaining »trapped« in the giant web of the biofilm. This mechanical entrapment lowers their concentration and antimicrobial activity, so their usefulness for chronic infections is doubtful (Isiklar et al. 1996).

New mechanisms of bacterial resistance against some antibiotics based on »quorum-sensing« signals are being discovered (Hentzer and Givskov 2003; Ehrlich et al. 2005).

Antibiotic-Loaded PMMA for Biofilm

Bacteria adhere much less to antibiotic-loaded PMMA in experiments *in vitro*: PMMA-gentamicin infects with inocula 60 times greater than plain PMMA (Oga et al. 1992), while it has been demonstrated that *Proteus* and *Pseudomona* adherence on PMMA-gentamicin is difficult (Chang and Merritt 1994). These experiments suggest that PMMA-gentamicin could be very useful for the treatment of chronic infections.

Recently good results have been published in clinical series of two-stage exchange using antibiotics in cement for reimplantation, but patients receiving no systemic antibiotics at all. Infection was healed in 34 of 38 total knee arthroplasties (89% healing; Hoad-Reddick et al. 2005) and in 100 out of 114 total hip arthroplasties (87% healing; Hoad-Reddick et al. 2005) when antibiotics were used only in the cement for reimplantation.

Intracellular Bacteria

Crisis of Classical Immune Mechanisms

Along the past two decades it has been demonstrated that, in many clinical infections, the »classical« immune mechanism of recruitment (fraction C5a of complement), bacterial opsonization (fraction C3b of complement), adherence to specific membrane receptors, phagocytosis and killing inside phagolysosomes does not work. In fact, many bacteria are able to survive inside cells (inside cytoplasm, endosomes, some vesicles or phagolyso-

somes) by different molecular mechanisms under adverse conditions.

Staphylococcus: Facultative Intracellular

Staphylococci may also live as a facultative intracellular. When surviving inside host cells they maintain defective oxidative mechanisms, this lowers metabolic activity, the result of which is a very slow growth, infrequent mitosis, and an ineffective membrane transport. All these phenotypic changes determine that these species form very small clusters or colonies when cultured in laboratory: this is the explanation for the denomination »small colony variant« (SCV; Maurin and Raoult 1994; Proctor et al. 1995).

Demonstration of Intracellular *Staphylococcus*

These intracellular *Staphylococci* have been demonstrated in vitro and in clinical studies.

Cultures of osteoblasts were infected by *S. aureus*; after several hours of incubation, bacteria were demonstrated inside osseous cells. Moreover, if osteoblasts were lised, *S. aureus* may infect other cells in the culture (Ellington et al. 2003).

Intracellular *S. aureus* inside periprosthetic fibroblasts were demonstrated in five patients with recidivant and recurrent total hip arthroplasty infections. They had been treated previously by one or more conventional treatments without success. Infection was healed in all of them by means of a 2-stage exchange without spacer plus intracellularly-efficient antibiotics (Sendi et al. 2006).

Antibiotics Ineffective for Intracellular Bacteria

Many antibiotics are not effective for intracellular bacteria because of different reasons. Betalactams are unable to penetrate inside phagocytes, so they are not useful for intracellular bacteria in chronic infections. Aminoglycosides (gentamicin, tobramycin) penetrate cells by pynocitosis (a typical active membrane transport), but as membrane transport is defective (because of low metabolism), intracellular levels are very low after antibiotic treatment (Maurin and Raoult 1994).

Doxiciclin, amikacin and pefloxacin are inactivated by the acid media of phagolysosomes (Maurin and Raoult 1994). Those antibiotics blocking bacterial metabolism (tetracyclines, amikacin, pefloxacin) are hardly useful because the bacterial metabolism is very low.

Antibiotics Efficient for Intracellular Bacteria

Rifampin presents an excellent intracellular activity because of elevated transport and activity in acid media; several papers confirm its usefulness in vitro (Zimmerli et al. 1998; Ellington et al. 2006) and in clinical infections (Barberán et al. 2006).

Fluoroquinolones (ciprofloxacin, ofloxacin, levofloxacin) acumulate inside cytoplasm and lysosomes, so they present a very good activity inside cells. Their clinical efficiency in orthopaedic infections is also published (Barberán et al. 2006; Rissing 1997).

Cotrimoxazol (trimethoprim-sulfamethoxazole) presents a good intracellular transportation and a great activity inside phagocytes. Their clinical efficiency was demonstrated in a series of infected total hip and knee arthroplasties with a 67% of healing after 6 months of oral treatment followed by an exchange in one-stage (Stein et al. 1998).

Clindamycin also presents an elevated intracellular activity, is more efficient as more precocious is used, and is resistant to the vegetative changes described for SCV *Staphylococci*. This drug has been employed with success in some series (Ellington et al. 2006; Cordero-Ampuero et al. 2007).

The macrolide antibiotics (azitromicin, claritromicin) also acumulate inside cytoplasm and lysosomes and present great activity inside phagocytes, but their spectrum of activity is usually not useful for orthopaedic infections.

Linezolid, the first oxazolidinone, also presents a strong activity, but side effects must be controlled (Soriano et al. 2007).

All theses antibiotics are effective for oral administration because they get a good avaibility, but

Table 13.1. Antibiotics efficient for intracellular bacteria

Class of antibiotic	Antibiotics
Inhibitor of nucleic acid	Rifampin
Fluoroquinolones	Ciprofloxacin Levofloxacin/ofloxacin
Antimetabolites	Trimethoprim/ sulphamethoxazole
Lincosamides	Clindamycin
Macrolides	Azitromicin Claritromicin
Oxazolidinone	Linezolid

at least some of them (rifampin and quinolones) must be used in combination to avoid development of resistances (Table 13.1).

Results in Clinical Infections in Orthopaedic Surgery

Some clinical series from European hospitals have been published for treatment of infected arthroplasties when considering the problem of intracellular bacteria.

The classical one of Drancourt, the first one published, applied a long combined oral antibiotherapy of rifampin plus ofloxacin for 6 months, followed by a surgery of one-stage exchange in unstable total hips and in all total knees. They obtained microbiological healing in 81% of hips and 69% of knees (Drancourt et al. 1993).

The group of Zimmerli has communicated a series of five infected hips by SCV *Staphylococcus aureus* demonstrated inside periprosthetic fibroblasts. Patients had been treated previously by conventional treatments without success. The five infections were healed by means of a two-stage exchange without spacer and with the use of intracellular-efficient antibiotics (Sendi et al. 2006).

We have recently published a clinical series about treatment of 40 chronic arthroplasty infections, 16 hips and 24 knees (Cordero-Ampuero et al. 2007). The series included 6 cases with polymicrobial isolates, 19 cases with methicillin-resistant *Staphylococcus* among 35 infections by these bacteria, and other infections by multirresistant and/or problematic Gram-negatives (4 *Enterococcus*, 2 *Pseudomonas*, 2 *Proteus*, 1 *Serratia*). Patients were treated with a combined strategy: two-stage exchange, reimplantation with PMMA-gentamicin-clindamycin, and 6 months of oral antibiotic therapy. A spacer was not used in hips; it was a static spacer model in knees (hand-made of PMMA-gentamicin-clindamycin). The reimplantation surgery was delayed until clinical and serological normalization. The oral therapy was a combination of antibiotics with activity inside biofilm and inside cells: rifampin, ofloxacin/levofloxacin, ciprofloxacin, cotrimoxazol, clindamycin, fosfomycin, linezolid with). After a mean follow-up of 4 years (2–9) the infection remained healed in 15/16 hips (93.8%) and in 23/24 knees (95.8%), while the orthopaedic results obtained an average Harris Hip Score of 94 (84-98) for hips and an average Knee Society Clinical Score of 83 (59-93) / 67 (30-90) for knees. Our good results support the use of this combined protocol.

Future

New strategies and many different ways have been and continue to be explored. Anti-»quorum-sensing« drugs and substances are among them (Kaufmann et al. 2008; Simonetti et al. 2008). Hypothetic future implants with incorporated automatic mechanisms to detect and treat bacteria have also been proposed (Ehrlich et al. 2005). For the moment, all of them continue to be investigational.

Among new antibiotics just launched in the market daptomycin and tygecyclin are the most interesting. Daptomycin, a lipopeptide, compares favourably with vancomycin in osteoarticular infections, but differences are non-significant. There is no published experience of tygecyclin for clinical osteoarticular infections.

Other antibiotics are to be commercialized in the very near future. Dalbavancin, a lipoglycopeptide, has the advantage of administration once a week because of its long half-life (9–12 days); it

presents a high bactericidal activity against methicillin-resistant *Staphylococci*. Ceftobiprole, the first beta-lactam active simultaneously against methicillin-resistant *Staphylococci* and against Gram-negatives (similar activity against Gram-negatives as 4th-generation cephalosporins), may be a promising substance.

References

Arizono T, Oga M, Sugioka Y (1992) Increased resistance of bacteria after adherence to polymethyl-metacrilate. An in vitro study. Acta Orthop Scand 63: 661–664

Barberán J, Aguilar L, Carroquino G, Giménez MJ, Sánchez B, Martínez D, Prieto J (2006) Conservative treatment of staphylococcal prosthetic joint infections in elderly patients. Am J Med 119: 993.e7–10

Chang CC, Merritt K (1994) Infection at the site of implanted materials with and without preadhered bacteria. J Orthop Res 12: 526–531

Chang CC, Merritt K (1994) Infection at the site of implanted materials with and without preadhered bacteria. J Orthop Res 12: 526–531

Cordero J (1999) Infection of orthopaedic implants. Theory and practice. European Instructional Course Lectures 165–173

Cordero J, Garcia-Cimbrelo E (2000) Mechanisms of bacterial resistance in implant infection. Hip International 10: 139–144

Cordero J, Munuera L, Folgueira MD (1994) Influence of metal implants on infection. J Bone Joint Surg (Br) 76-B: 717–720

Cordero J, Munuera L, Folgueira MD (1996) Influence of bacterial strains on bone infection. J Orthop Res 14: 663–667

Cordero-Ampuero J (2000) Mecanismos de resistencia bacteriana en la infección de implantes. Rev Orthop Traum 44: 115–126

Cordero-Ampuero J, Esteban J, García-Cimbrelo E, Munuera L, Escobar R (2007) Low relapse with oral antibiotics plus two-stage exchange for late arthroplasty infections in 40 patients after 2-to-9 years. Acta Orthop 78: 511–519

Crockarell JR, Hanssen AD, Osmon DR, Morrey BF (1998) Treatment of infection with débridement and retention of the components following hip arthroplasty. J Bone Joint Surg (Am) 80-A: 1306–1313

Donlan RM (2001) Biofilm formation: a clinically relevant microbiological process. Clin Inf Dis 33: 1387–1392

Drancourt M, Stein A, Argenson JN, Zannier A, Curvale G, Raoult D (1993) Oral rifampin plus ofloxacin for treatment of staphylococcus-infected orthopedic implants. Antimicrob Agents Chemother 37: 1214–1218

Ehrlich GD, Stoodley P, Kathju S et al. (2005) Engineering approaches for the detection and control of orthopaedic biofilm infections. Clin Orthop 437: 59–66

Ellington JK, Harris M, Hudson MC, Vishin S, Webb LX, Sherertz R (2006) Intracellular Staphylococcus aureus and antibiotic resistance: implications for treatment of staphylococcal osteomyelitits. J Orthop Res 24: 87–93

Ellington JK, Harris M, Webb L, Smith B, Smith T, Tan K, Hudson M (2003) Intracellular Staphylococcus aureus. A mechanism for the indolence of osteomyelitis. J Bone Joint Surg (Br) 85: 918–921

Esteban J, Gómez-Barrena E, Cordero J, Zamora N, Kinnari TJ, Fernández-Roblas R (2008) Evaluation of quantitative cultures from sonicated retrieved orthopaedic implants in the diagnosis of orthopaedic infection. J Clin Microbiol 46: 488–492

Fischer B, Vaudaux P, Magnin M, Mestikawy YE, Proctor RA, Lew DP, Vasey H (1996) Novel animal model for studying the molecular mechanisms of bacterial adhesion to bone-implanted metallic devices: role of fibronectin in staphylococcus aureus adhesion. J Orthop Res 14: 914–920

Garvin KL, Hanssen AD (1995) Infection after Total Hip Arthroplasty. J Bone Joint Surg (Am) 77-A: 1576–1588

Gristina AG, Costerton JW (1985) Bacterial adherence to biomaterials and tissue. J Bone Joint Surg (Am) 67-A: 264–273

Gristina AG, Naylor PT, Myrvik QN (1991) Mechanisms of Musculoskeletal Sepsis. Orthop Clin North Am 22: 363–371

Hentzer M, Givskov M (2003) Pharmacological inhibition of quorum sensing for the treatment of chronic bacterial infections. J Clin Invest 112: 1300–1307

Hoad-Reddick DA, Evans CR, Norman P, Stockley I (2005) Is there a role for extended antibiotic therapy in a two-stage revision of the infected knee arthroplasty? J Bone Joint Surg (Br) 87-B: 171–175

Isiklar ZU, Darouiche RO, Landon GC, Beck T (1996) Efficacy of antibiotics alone for orthopaedic device related infections. Clin Orthop 332: 184–189

Kaufmann GF, Park J, Janda KD (2008) Bacterial quorum sensing: a new target for anti-infective immunotherapy. Expert Opin Biol Ther 8: 719–724

Maurin M, Raoult D (1994) Phagolysosomal alkalinization and intracellular killing of staphylococcus aureus by amikacin. J Infect Dis 169: 330–336

Mihalko WM, Manaswi A, Cui Q, Parvizi J, Schmalzried TP, Saleh KJ (2008) Diagnosis and treatment of the infected primary total knee arthroplasty. AAOS Instr Course Lect 57: 327–339

Oga M, Arizono T, Sugioka Y (1992) Inhibition of bacterial adhesion by tobramycin-impregnated PMMA bone cement. Acta Orthop Scand 63: 301–304

Petty W (1978) The effect of methylmethacrylate on chemotaxis of polymorphonuclear leukocytes. J Bone Joint Surg (Am) 60-A: 492–498

Petty W, Spanier S, Shuster JJ, Silverthorne C (1985) The influence of skeletal implants on incidence of infection. J Bone Joint Surg (Am) 67-A: 1236–1244

Proctor RA, van Langevelde P, Kristjansson M, Maslow JN, Arbeit RD (1995) Persistent and relapsing infections associated with small-colony variants of staphylococcus aureus. Clin Infect Dis 20: 95–102

Rissing JP (1997) Antimicrobial therapy for chronic osteomyelitis in adults: role of the quinolones. Clin Infect Dis 25: 1327–1333

Sendi P, Rohrbach M, Graber P, Frei R, Ochsner PE, Zimmerli W (2006) Staphylococcus aureus small colony variants in prosthetic joint infection. Clin Infect Dis 43: 961–967

Simonetti O, Cirioni O, Ghiselli R et al. (2008) RNAIII-inhibiting peptide enchances healing of wounds infected with methicillin-resistant Staphylococcus aureus. Antimicrob Agents Chemother 52: 2205–2211

Soriano A, Gómez J, Gómez L, Azanza JR, Pérez R, Romero F, Pons M, Bella F, Velasco M, Mensa J (2007) Efficacy and tolerability of prolonged linezolid therapy in the treatment of orthopedic implant infections. Eur J Clin Microbiol Infect Dis 26: 353–356

Stein A, Bataille JF, Drancourt M, Curvale G, Argenson JN, Groulier P, et al. (1998) Ambulatory treatment of multidrug-resistant Staphylococcus-infected ortohopedic implants with high-dose oral co-trimoxazole (trimethoprim-sulfamethoxazole). Antimicrob Agents Chemother 42: 3086–3091

Stockley I, Mockford BJ, Hoad-Reddick A, Norman P (2008) The use of two-stage exchange arthroplasty with depot antibiotics in the absence of long-term antibiotic therapy in infected total hip replacement. J Bone Joint Surg (Br) 90: 145–148

Trampuz A, Piper KE, Jacobson MJ et al. (2007) Sonication of removed hip and knee prostheses for diagnosis of infection. N Engl J Med 357: 654–663

Zimmerli W, Widmer AF, Blatter M, Frei R, Ochsner PE (1998) Role of rifampin for treatment of orthopedic implant-related staphylococcal infections: a randomized controlled trial. Foreign-Body Infection (FBI) Study Group. JAMA 279: 1537–1541

Introduction: Revision Cemented Versus Uncemented

Philipp Lubinus

In the long run man-made devices are bound to fail.

In the case of implants for arthroplasty the failure can happen due to mechanical reasons like wear and breakage of an implant or due to biological reasons like infection and destruction of the very bone which sustains the implants fixation.

The probably most important mechanism of implant-loosening consists of a mechanical cause and its biological response.

Wear at the bearing surfaces and abrasive processes at the implants surface to the bone generate continually a huge number of microscopic and submicroscopic non-biodegradable particles, which are small enough to travel quite a distance in the biological environment.

These very small and many particles consist either of polyethylene from a conventional bearing or of methylmetacrylat from a cemented implants fixation or are eventually particles of metal from a hard bearing or an implants surface and all of them are provoking an inflammatory biological response.

Macrophages unavailingly trying to digest these particles induce a cascade of cytokines, enzymes and growth factors thus activating the periprosthetic tissues resulting in the formation of osteolytic lesions or granulomas.

As these granulomas increase in size over time and are eating up more and more bone stock, the implants fixation to the bone becomes progressively compromised, leading in the end to either periprosthetic fracture or loosening of the implant.

The type and size of the bone loss is the surgeons major concern after failed arthroplasty implants, because big bone loss can make it much harder to obtain a good long-term fixation for the revision implant.

In order to not take too much fun out of the following controversial presentations I would like to present just a few thoughts about the different advantages and disadvantages of cemented and cementless revisions:

Experience with cemented reconstructions out of the last decades have shown that their durability is not always flawless and especially in cases with major bone loss the longevity of cemented reconstructions is not always satisfying, and if they fail, you will have more bone deficiencies than before the last revision.

On the other hand, there are for sure some good reasons to use antibiotics loaded bone cement in the case of septic revisions, as you can generate very high levels of antibacterial potency right at the front line with little systemic risks and good primary stability.

The bigger the bone loss and the younger the patient the more important reconstruction of bone stock becomes, what is favorably achieved by using bone transplants or substitutes and cementless implants.

Smaller loss of bone stock in an elderly patient until today gives a good indication for a cemented revision.

Maybe the combination of transplanted bone and cement as used following Exeter or Ullmark technique closes the gap between strictly cemented and cementless techniques nicely.

Cemented revision THA

Libor Luňáček

Introduction

Revision total hip arthroplasty generally represents a challenge even for the experienced surgeon. We are facing with the compromised bone and soft-tissue situation that frequently may affect the long-term results of the revision. The results achieved after the replacement of total hip arthroplasty by another cemented implant under specific conditions in aseptic and septic failure of THAs may be successful. Preoperative bone loss and cement technique at the time of revision surgery can affect the long-term durability of a cemented revision following loosening. Very important is ability of cemented revisions forming a lasting microinterlock with the endosteal surface of bone (DeLee and Charnley 1976; Krbec et al. 1992).

Material and Methods

In the period from 2000 to 2006, 393 aseptic revision surgeries of total hip arthroplasty were performed at the author's departement. In 2003–2006 we performed two-stage reimplantation with classical molded cement spacer in the treatment of 25 patients with potencially infected THA and we compared results with the first group. In aseptic revision group the indication for operation was loosening of degree II or III of the classification according to Krbec et al. The surgery was performed from the Watson-Jones or Bauer approach. The clinical condition was evaluated on the basis of the Harris Hip Score and a radiograph was made to monitor changes in the position of the cup, linear wear, the presence and size of the radiolucent zone. The cemented revision THA was always done with the use of antibiotic-containing cement.

At the authors' department we reviewed a group of 69 patients (57 women, 12 men) with the cemented cup replaced by another cemented cup and the original femoral monocomponent with the 32 mm head diameter the surface of which was not damaged was left in place. The indication for operation was loosening of degree II or III of the classification according to Krbec et al. (1992). The surgery was performed from the Watson-Jones or Bauer approach. The cup was always revised with the use of antibiotic-containing cement by the second-generation cementing technique. Augmentation was used in 11 cups. The original femoral component was always returned to the original cemented bed and a cement mantle was added in the proximal part in 15 patients. Poldi-Čech cups were replaced in all patients of the followed-up cohort (63 times loosening – 91%, 6 times breakage – 9%). At revision surgery 3 types of cups were used (Poldi-Čech – 44 times, Ultima – 20

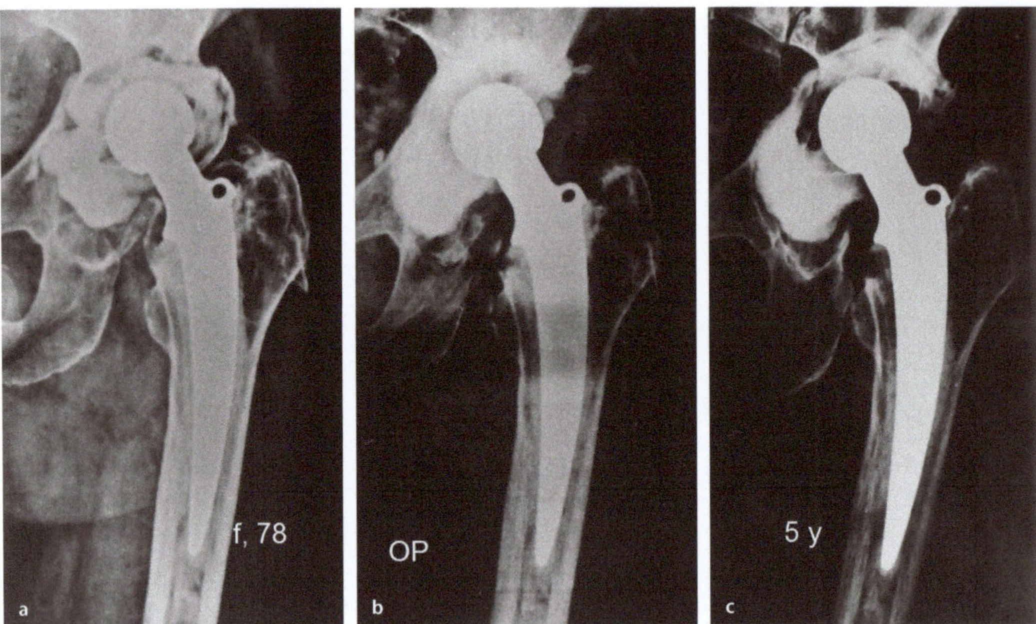

Fig. 15.1a–c. Radiographs of a 78-year-old female patient: **a** a loosening and destruction of the cup 14 years after total hip arthroplasty, **b** after revision: a cemented cup (bulk filling with cement and additional cementing of the femoral component, **c** a follow-up radiograph after 5 years with a finding of a radiolucent line in the medial part of the cup cement

times, SPC – 5 times). The results were evaluated in 48 patients (40 women, 8 men) with the average interval of 63 months after revision of the cup (range, 46–112 months). However, the clinical and radiograph evaluation of the condition was made only in 45 patients.

The Harris Hip Score was on average 78 points (range 51–97 points). Radiographs did not show any change in the position of the cup. The linear wear up to 1 mm was revealed in 4 cups and above 1 mm in 1 cup (11% of the evaluated patients). The radiolucent line in zone III according to DeLee and Charnley was present in 4 cups, in zones II and III in another 4 cups, i.e. in total in 8 of 45 cups (18%). The group of 45 followed-up patients may be considered a sufficiently representative sample of the original 69-member cohort (minimally 7 patients died in the follow-up period, 3 patients were not included in the evaluation). With regard to the average follow-up of 63 months the results may be considered as medium-term.

The average interval between primary total hip arthroplasty and revision of 130 months is compa-rable with the results of similar studies by other authors. The results of the clinical evaluation on the basis of Harris Hip Score are not convincing (range 51–97 points, and average 78 points). Radiographs showed a radiolucent zone in 8 cups (18 %; Fig. 15.1). Another 3 patients were at the time of evaluation after a repeated revision of the cup for loosening (at the interval of 22 to 34 months). The evaluation of other patients of the followed-up cohort, however, produced rather unconvincing results.

Discussion

In certain cases it concerns mainly older patients with a changed shape of the acetabulum where, however, the structure was preserved and implantation of the cementless cup, if necessary with the application of bone grafts, may cause in older patients a number of problems (life-threatening bleeding immediately after the surgery, delayed os-teointegration of bone grafts requiring a long-term

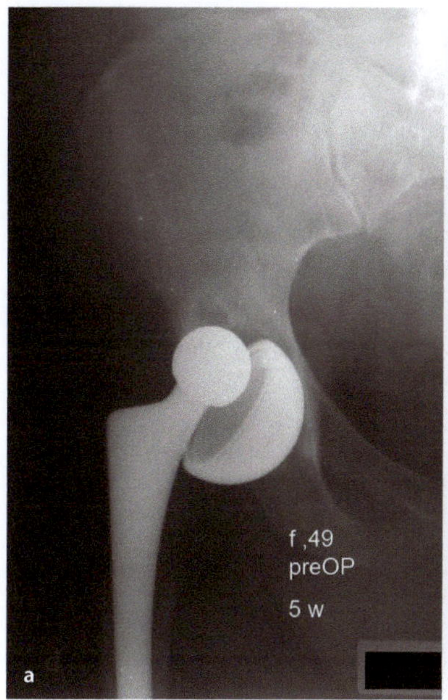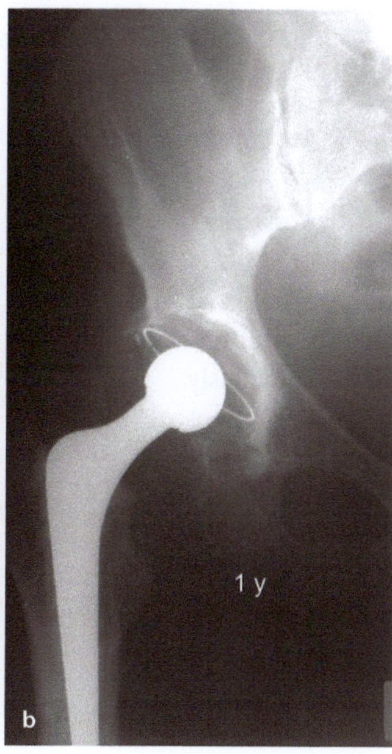

Fig. 15.2a,b. Radiographs of a 49-year-old female patient: **a** A cup loosening 5 weeks after primary cementless total hip arthroplasty; **b** after revision: a cemented THA with standard components

non-weight-bearing of the extremity). The application of a cemented component even with a thicker cement mantle (»LORR cement«) is convenient in cases where these patient expects from the surgery mainly pain relief.

Femoral reconstruction in the revision technique rely on fixation to healthy diaphyseal bone and is favorably compared with the second-generation cementing technique. In the face of severe bone loss, the most important issue is to restore or augment the bone stock, and impaction grafting has been a popular option (Slooff et al. 1993), but we have not any experience with them. Bone quality and patient age also appear to be important factors in predicting the success with a cemented revision stem. The use of longer stems is better to obtain these improved results, at least 10 cm beyond the femoral defect (Breusch and Malchau 2005). Recently described techniques in which revision stems are cemented into impacted cancellous allograft appear promising (Schreurs et al. 2001). The results with cemented femoral revision stems with the application of second-generation cementing techniques improved results markedly, with loosening rates of 10% at 10 years in a number of series.

The cement-within-cement technique is indeed not a new technique (Eftekhar in 1978). Removal of all foreign material is the normal practice at the time of revision arthroplasty. However, removal of well fixed bone cement is time consuming, can result in significant bone stock loss and increases the risk of femoral shaft perforation or fracture. The indications for the use of the cement-within-cement technique include a broken stem with an intact distal cement mantle, the temporary removal of a femoral component for revision of a loose cup to improve exposure, conversion from a cemented hemiarthroplasty to a THA, recurrent dislocation secondary to component malposition, and poor integration or failure of the cementless femoral komponent (Fig. 15.2).

In revision for sepsis we do recommend removal of all old cement mantle, there is only one report in literature with results of two-stage revision hip arthroplasty with retention of well-fixed femoral component mantle. Authors referred that no patients were suspected of having a recurrence of infection (Blake et al. 2008).

In acetabular reconstruction any revision acetabular component must optimize the use of whatever bone remains after primary hardware is removed. The Paprosky classification of acetabular bone deficiency in revision hip arthroplasty seems to be an appropriate measure to use, we are using our classification according to Krbec et al. (1992). Cemented components for revision fixation are used either with acetabular reconstruction cages or with impaction grafting techniques (Koudela and Malotín 2001; Slooff et al. 1993; Schreurs et al. 2001). For patients with the pelvic discontinuity type of THA failure, there are no obviously superior methods of reconstruction. The treatment revision options for these patients include antiprotrusio cages and cemented cups, or plate augmentation with cemented or cementless cups. The amount of bone support that is present in the ilium is a critical factor for the resulting stability of the patient's acetabular component. If the bone loss is greater than use of an allografts must be considered (Schreurs et al. 2001; Berry and Müller 1992).

Conclusion

A good integration of the cemented implant used in revision was evident only in cases of a perfectly preserved acetabulum ad femur both from the viewpoint of shape and structure. Bone removal at the time of the initial implantation of the stem and bone loss due to subsequent failure of the implant left little intramedullary cancellous bone, which may cause anchoring of cemented implant problematic and explain the higher rate of loosening observed.

The evaluation of other patients of the followed-up cohort, however, produced rather unconvincing results. The application of a cemented component with a thicker cement mantle is convenient in cases where the patient expects from the surgery mainly pain relief. In septic cases we prefer bone cement with combination of the antibiotics gentamicin and clindamycin, which is known to have a synergistic bactericidal effect on more than 90% of the bacteria common to infected arthroplasty cases. Advantages of using cemented implants is immediate fixation attainment, for using in primary septic cases (septic coxitis; ☐ Fig. 15.3), and is appropriate for elderly patiens and patiens with good bone stock.

☐ **Table 15.1.** Advantages of cemented revision – Summary

I	Performs well in all age groups
II	Provided good results in good indications
III	Immediate fixation attained, appropriate for elderly patients and patients with good bone stock
IV	Local antibiotic delivery carrier – antibiotic-loaded cement
V	Possibility add extra antibiotic [Vancomycin]
VI	Biologic reconstruction with impaction grafting for acetabulum
VII	Cement-in-cement technique in aseptic cases for femoral component

Very important is careful preoperative planning, we have to answer the following questions: What is the cause of failure? Is there bone loss? What kind of primary fixation? Remaining bone stock enough to anchor a new implant? Only one component exchange? Can we use standard component? In a cup revision we recommend use of cemented implant in situations with no large bone defects, try to expose bleeding cancellous bone if possible, use jet lavage, cages with cement or bone grafts. On the femoral side in some cases we use cement-within-cement technique. This procedure is not possible in cases with enormous bone lost and large defects. The stem must to be anchored at least 8 to 10 cm deep in healthy bone. In septic cases we do remove all old cement mantle. Our cemented indications are: aseptic loosening with good bone stock, septic hip in problematic cases (users, immunodeficiency, haematologic), elderly patiens.

Revision of a failed THA with use of cement provided good result in good indications, the rate of loosening at the time medium follow-up seems to be in some articles higher than that commonly reported after revision with use of uncemented implants (Breusch and Malchau 2005; Langlais 2003; Gie et al. 1993). There are a multitude of problems that have to be individually resolved in each patient.

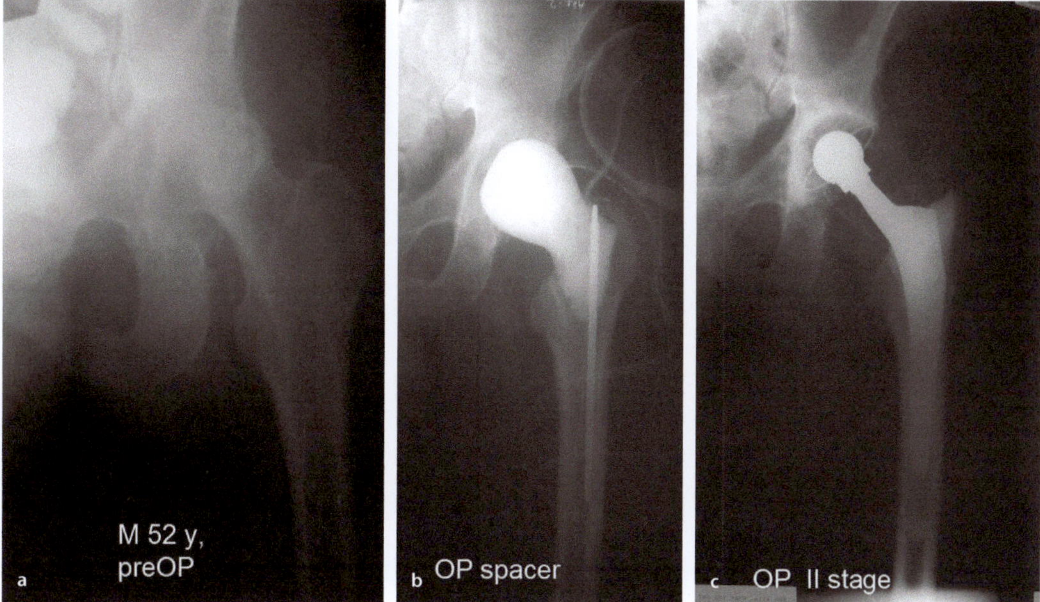

Fig. 15.3a–c. Radiographs of a 52-year-old male patient: **a** Purulent coxitis with destruction, **b** GEA and cemented spacer with AB loaded bone cement, c – after revision: the cemented THA was implanted after 8 weeks

References

Berry DJ, Müller ME (1992) Revision arthroplasty using an anti-protrusio cage for massive acetabular deficiency. J Bone Joint Surg Br 74-B: 711–715

Blake SM, Hubble MJ, Howell JR, Timperley AJ, Gie GA (2008) Results of in-cement revision of infected total hip arthroplasty. J Bone Joint Surg B Volume 90B (Suppl II): 297–298

Breusch S, Malchau H (2005) The well-cemented total hip arthroplasty. Springer, Berlin Heidelberg New York Tokyo

DeLee JG, Charnley J (1976) Radiological demarcation of cemented sockets in total hip replacement. Clin Orthop 121: 20–32

Gie GA, Linder L, Ling RS, Simon JP, Slooff TJ, Timperley AJ (1993) Impacted cancellous allografts and cement for revision total hip arthroplasty. J Bone Joint Surg Br 75-B: 14–21

Koudela K, Malotín T (2001) Rekonstrukce acetabula při výměně asepticky uvolněné jamky. Acta Chir Orthop Traum čech 68: 162–167

Krbec M, Čech O, Džupa V (1992) Reoperace totální endoprotézy kyčelního kloubu – diagnostika a RTG klasifikace. Acta Chir Orthop Traum čech 59: 23–26

Langlais F (2003) Can we improve the results of revision arthroplasty for infected total hip replacement? J Bone Joint Surg [Br] 85-B: 637–640

Paprosky WG, Perona PG, Lawrence JM (1994) Acetabular defect classification and surgical reconstruction in revision arthroplasty: a 6-year follow-up evaluation. J Arthroplasty 9: 33–44

Quinlan JF, O'Shea K, Doyle F, Brady OH (2006) In-cement technique for revision hip arthroplasty. J Bone Joint Surg Br 88: 730–733

Raut VV, Siney PD, Wroblevski BM (1995) Cemented revision for aseptic acetabular loosening. J Bone Joint Surg 77-B: 357–36l

Schreurs BW, Arts JJ, Verdonschot N, Buma P, Slooff TJ, Gardeniers JW (2005) Femoral component revision with use of impaction bone-grafting and a cemented polished stem. J Bone Joint Surg Am 87-A: 2499–2507

Schreurs BW, Slooff TJJ, Gardeniers JWM, Buma P (2001) Acetabular reconstruction with bone impaction grafting and a cemented cup: 20 years' experience. Clin Orthop 393: 202–215

Slooff TJ, Schimmel JW, Buma P (1993) Cement fixation with bone grafts. Orthop Clin North Am 24: 667–677

Pro Uncemented Revision

Martin Krbec

Introduction

It is little bit confusing to compare cemented and non-cemented principles in terms of survival rate in hip replacements without further specification of the non-cemented implant, nor in primary neither in revision surgery. Considering many different factors which can influence the integration of the bone to the implant surface in non-cemented implants, as far as material used, roughness of the surface, shape of the cup and stem and biomechanical principles of fixation, it is necessary to compare these modalities in different non-cemented types in the first instance amongst each other. Great development occurred during the time since the beginning of massive introduction of non-cemented implantations in late eighties. Then, the successful non-cemented systems could be compared against the cemented ones, which were considered as safe and successful, mainly through the follow-ups in THR registries. Looking at the literature, there are some articles describing comparison of outcomes of cemented and non-cemented hips (Iorio et al. 2008; Templeton et al. 2001; Weber et al. 1996; Haydon et al. 2004), but these articles are mainly level 3 or 4 of evidence studies or some metaanalyses. There is hardly possible to perform randomised double-blind controlled study on this topic. In this paper we focused on some findings from the literature confirming the efficacy of non-cemented revision surgery. Based on data describing non-cemented aseptic revisions and with references from the literature and own experience we introduce our concept of non-cemented revision even in infected THR.

Material and Methods

There are very successfully cemented implants with long-term survival according to the registers (Swedish Hip Arthroplasty Register 2007; Norwegian Arthroplasty Register 2008), as e.g. Charnley prosthesis with more then 30 years survival rate, Exeter hip, Müller banana stem, Lubinus etc. On the other hand, we recorded even in the past 15 years very unhappy attempts to ameliorate the shape and biomechanic features of the cemented prosthesis, which ended with catastrophical outcomes after several years, as e.g. use of an acrylic head, the introduction of CF-30 type etc. The shape of the stem, the finish of the surface and material used play a role in survival rate even in cemented implants.

In cemented THA the interface bone-cement is just from the time point of implantation under active remodelation. At the beginning, the shrinking of the cement layer occurs which is followed by haematoma-building and organizing and within a couple of weeks the remodelation of the bone is in progress. Later, the fixation of the cement to the bone develops in firm stabilisation of the cement sheath. This is dependent on the shape and surface of the implant and responding to the transmission of the forces from the implant through the cement mantle to the bone.

Cemented fixation, both in primary and revision THA suppose to be stable and durable under these conditions:

1. the bony contact surface should have spongious structure,
2. the cement layer should be of appropriate and regular thickness around the stem and should spread entirely the preformed bony bed,
3. no major bone defects should be present. Even minor defect cause irregular thickness of the cement layer with an influence on the biomechanics and survival of the fixation.

In revision surgery there are usually one or mostly all these conditions violated.

Particularly in revision surgery with loosening of the implant we record usually the surface of the bony bed formed by cortical glabrous bone and of irregular shape of the cavity. Even in use of greater amount of cement according to the principle filling of the defects on the acetabular side as well as on the femoral side, the proper integration of bone and cement could not be expected.

There is usual statement heard from the cement popularizers that no uncemented implant provides as excellent results as cemented ones mentioned above.

This is partially true, but analyzing this statement, we should take in consideration, that the history of widely used non-cemented THR is about 15 years younger if we do not take in account the McKee and Farrar type and others similar types.

There were many false routes followed during the development, concerning mainly the shape and geometry of the implants, the material with not enough potential to provide good osteointegration, the roughness and structure of the surface. This handicap of the non-cemented implants is nowadays run down and modern cementless implants with rough active titanium surface and with press-fit mechanism of anchorage or by use of conic threaded cup, or combined proximal and distal fixation of the stem, and also HA-coating provide excellent long-term results for more then 20 years of successful survival. This principle and effect is widely applied also in revision surgery in recent years. Considering the infected hip arthroplasty, there are different situations according to the type and onset of the infection which should be taken in account. But the decision-making whether to use cemented or non-cemented arthroplasty (Sanchez-Sotelo et al. 2008) is based mainly on the ground philosophy of the hip surgery mentioned above. In our opinion, the role of antibiotic-impregnated cement in elimination of the infection is seen more in the effect of antibiotic-loaded cement spacer during the implant-free period as a part of two-stage revision rather then in cementing of components. Recently, in the literature there is also mentioned successful one-stage non-cemented revision in infected hip (Yoo et al. 2008).

Results

In case of infected THR, there are several different possibilities of the treatment according to the type and onset of infection, presence of potential loosening of the implant and according to the usual tactics of revision, namely if one- or two-stage procedure is proposed.

In case of early infection, within the first two or three weeks after primary implantation, the revision of cemented implant with its preservation is performed together with debridement and necrectomy, and only the non-fixed components as head is replaced. In case of non-cemented implant there is the possibility to replace the whole prosthesis, as it is not yet usually integrated within such a short period. This could be considered as advantage in order to diminish the risk of persistent infection.

Table 16.1. Advantages of non- cemented implants of the hip joint in revision surgery. The preferences of indication are extremely regional-dependent

	Non-cemented	Cemented
Duration of Surgery	Quicker procedure	Longer due to cement hardening
Technical Demand on surgery	Less demanding surgery	Demanding on cementing technique and bone defects management
Technical Demand on implant construction	More sophisticated	More simple
Mode of primary fixation	Mostly press-fit	Cement mantle between bone and implant
Mode of secondary Fixation	Direct bone ingrowth, according to the surface	Bone remodelation on contact surface with cement
Durability of fixation, survival	Comparable to the cemented or better	Comparable
Extraction feasibility	Worse then cemented	Simple, cement extraction is time consuming
Usability in osteoporotic terrain	Worse then cemented	Better then uncemented
Regional preference	North America, Australia, East Asia, Austria	Scandinavia, partially northern Europe
Use in young active patients	Preferable	Regionally different
Price	More expensive	Less expensive
Feasibility and durability for revision surgery	More suitable and durable	Less durable
Feasibility for revision in infection	Better, with antibiotic impregnated resorbable scaffold	Worse, need for mechanically less resistent antibiotics-loaded cement

In case of so-called delayed or subacute infection (onset from two months to 1 year after primary surgery), the whole implant removal is necessary, as there is usually glycocalix present on the implant surface. The removal is relatively easy in cemented hips, with careful removal of the cement, which is usually less or more loose. Also the removal of non-cemented hip is in this type of infection relatively easy as the osteointegration is usually violated due to bacterial activity, but sometimes the fixation is firm and stable enough and the explantation could be rather problematic.

In case of one-stage revision the use of cemented implants with antibiotics-loaded cement is preferred by some authors. The integration of the cement to the bone could be problematic, as described above. The use of bone grafts (bone bank) increase the risk of infection recurrency. In our opinion, the non-cemented implantation with the use of special revision implant is preferable, using two-stage procedures. Moreover, the local distribution of antibiotics is provided by use of antibiotics-loaded foam or gel. The two-stage revision seems to be rather safer from this point of view (Fink et al. 2008; Kraay et al. 2005).

The third type of situation which could follow is late, mainly hematogenous infection. In that case usually the implants are not loose. The attempt to perform revision with implant preservation and with exchange of only modular parts is possible if the diagnosis is done within days after its onset.

If there is a delay in diagnostics and course of the disease, the removal of the implant is necessary, what is simple but laborious in cemented types and very complicated in non-cemented types. The tactics of reimplantation is similar as in the case of early infection, one- or two-stage procedure. In one-stage procedure the presence of antibiotics-impregnated cement is considered as safety increasing measure. In our protocol if we once remove the implant, the two-stage revision surgery with use of non-cemented implants after 3-months period with antibiotics-loaded cement spacer is preferred (Kraay et al. 2005).

Based on this experience in our protocol the revision surgery of aseptic loosening is performed mainly with non-cemented implants. In case of the presence of acetabular or femoral defects, special revision implants could be used, which are able to provide excellent primary stability and can create also long-term integration of the implant.

In great defects we use routinely a Burch-Schneider reinforcement plate together with bone grafting and cemented cup. However, this construct should be considered more as non-cemented implantation. Rarely, we use big reconstruction cups as LOR, which is also considered in the literature as successful implant (Götze et al. 2003).

On the femoral side we prefer in all circumstances non-cemented implants with primary stability provided by fluted stem or by long enough stems with sharp cants. By using these implants we can expect the rebuilding and remodelation of the defects of proximal femur. Cemented stem in revision surgery is nowadays almost abandoned in our material. The same philosophy is applied in infected revisions in our hands. Two-stage procedure is preferred, with wide debridement and necrectomy in the first step; an antibiotic-loaded individual cement spacer is then inserted for the period of minimum 6 weeks. Systemic antibiotherapy is also performed. Then, as a second stage, new endoprosthesis is implanted with respect to the local conditions, in the same way as in aseptic loosening. The main goal is to obtain primary stability of the implant and to handle potential bone defects.

Discussion

Based on well-documented long-term follow-up, cementless fixation in primary hip replacement as well as in revision surgery seems to be as effective in long-term outcomes as cemented ones or even more in terms of survival. The polyethylene wear, which was considered by some authors as major disadvantage in non-cemented cups, is diminished by use of other pairing, like highly crosslinked PE and metal, or ceramic head and PE or even ceramics on ceramics. Also, in THR registries, such as in the Norwegian and Danish, even in the Swedish one (Swedish Hip Arthroplasty Register 2007; Norwegian Arthroplasty Register 2008; Danish Hip Arthroplasty Register 2007), there are recorded long-term trends of increase of numbers of non-cemented implantations in the past 5 years, both in primary and revision surgery.

In case of loosening of the implant, the disadvantage of bony defects and smooth inner cortical surface of the bone in the femoral cavity as well as in acetabulum, followed by irregular thickness of the cement layer, can influence the durability of the fixation and stability if cemented implant is used. Interdigitation of the cement into rough spongious bone surface as in primary surgery cannot be obtained. The cemented revision in the presence of the bony defects is possible and effective to perform only by use of the method of impaction grafting.

Following all these reasons we prefer in our protocol to use non-cemented implants even in infected revision THR. As we apply mainly a two-stage revision protocol in infected hip, we can abandon the potential advantage of the use of antibiotics-loaded cement, which represents only local antibiotics release in surrounding tissue. This effect is potentially obtained also by the use of antibiotic-loaded foam during shorter postoperative periods.

Of course, there are certain but rare conditions where we prefer cemented revision in our two-stage procedures, namely on acetabular side.

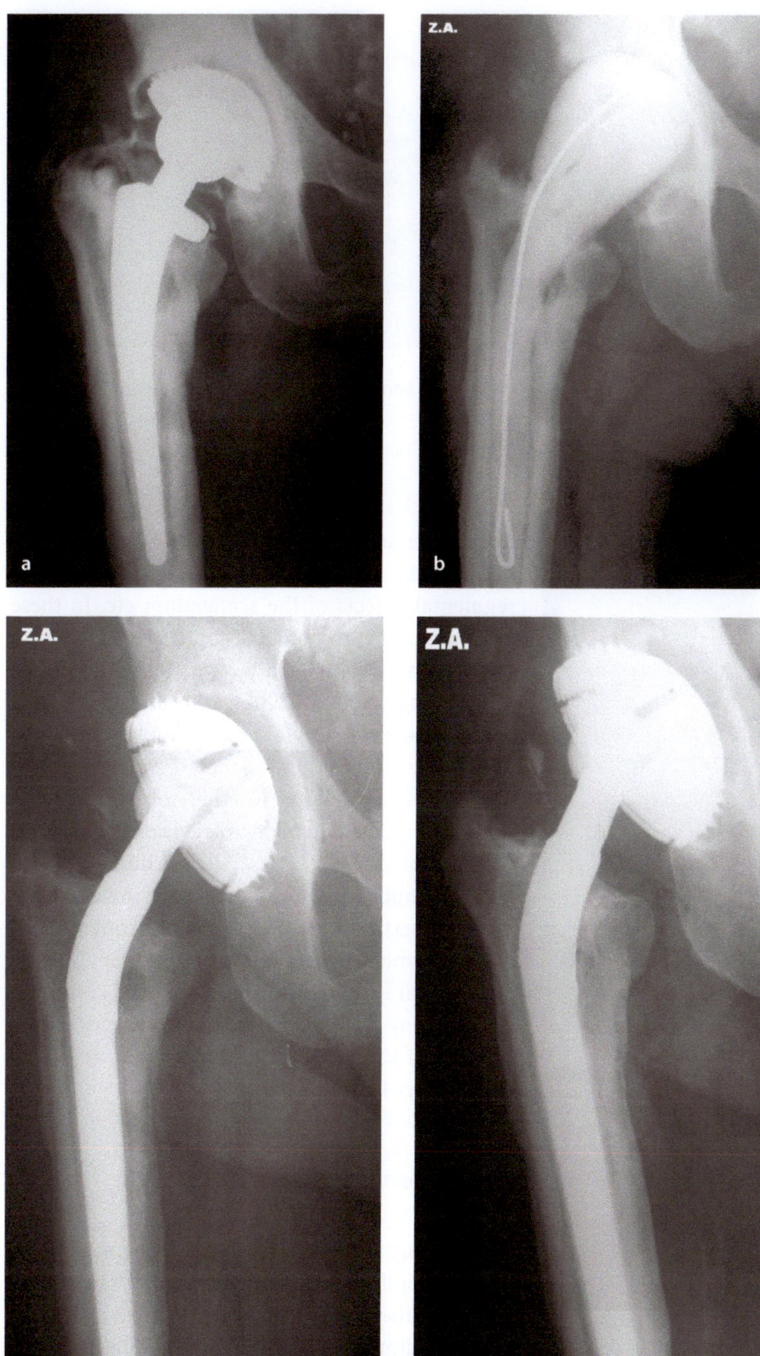

Fig. 16.1. a Hybrid THR showing delayed chronic infection with loosening of both components. **b** Cement spacer with antibiotics individually is inserted for 6 or more weeks. c New non-cemented THR with conventional cup and special revision stem inserted. **d** Outcome after 3 years. Good integration and stability of the implants

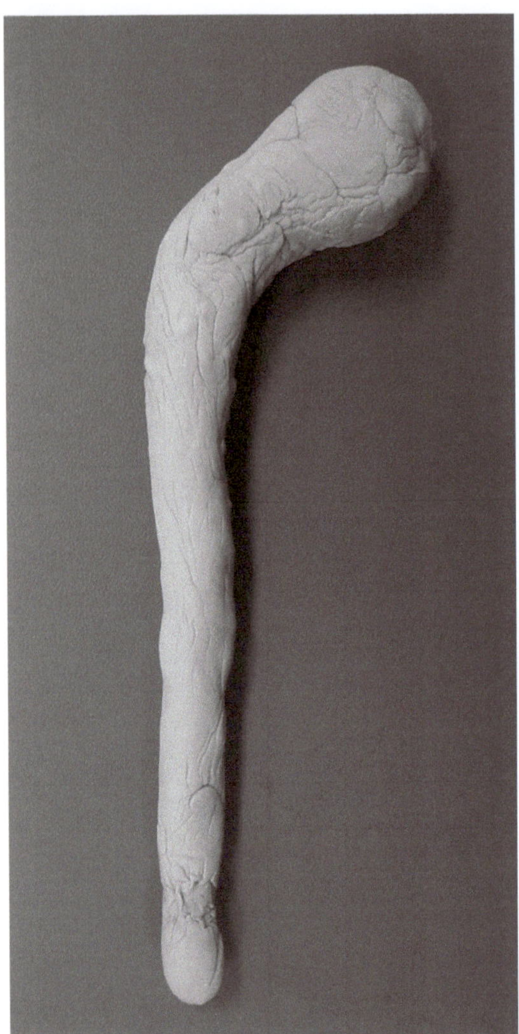

Fig. 16.2. Hand-formed individual spacer made from antibiotics-loaded cement

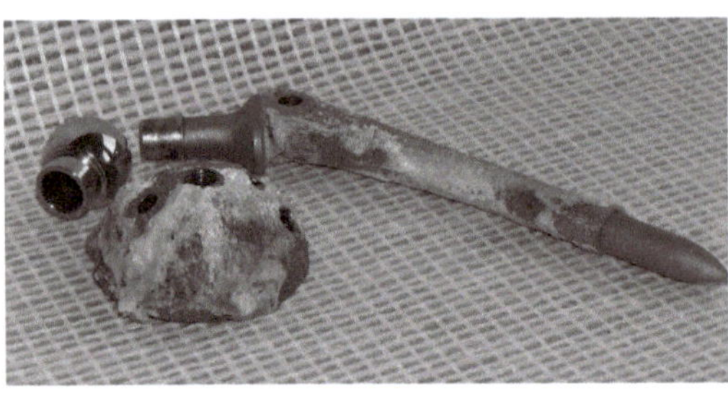

Fig. 16.3. Good signs of bone formation and integration of non-cemented implants (after removal)

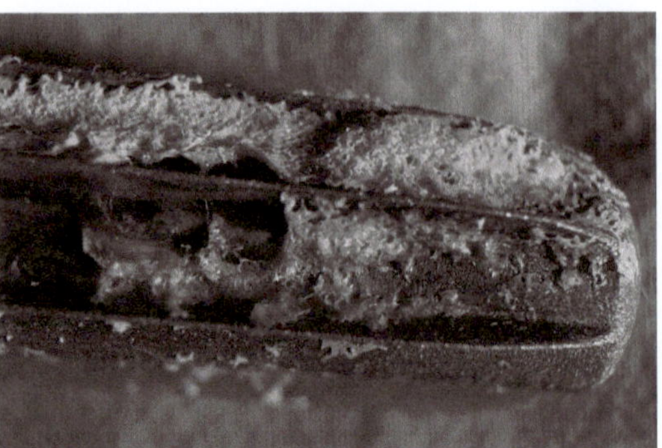

Fig. 16.4. Bony integration of special revision stem (after removal)

These are: inadequate quality of bone stock in the bedside, particularly substantial osteoporosis, segmental defects of the acetabulum etc. In these cases we prefer to combine grafting with the use of bone chips completed with metal reinforement (Koudela and Malotín 2001), according to the local conditions, from simple metallic net together with cement layer up to Burch-Schneider plate.

In decision-making whether to use cemented or non-cemented implant in revision surgery we are motivated to obtain excellent primary stability which is under usual circumstances much easier by the insertion of a non-cemented conventional or non-cemented special revision implant. There are very rare situations, where the local condition of the bony bed during revision surgery is the same or of similar worth as by primary implantation (Figs. 16.1–16.5).

Conclusion

Infected hip arthroplasty seems to be a very serious complication which can very dramatically influence the result of the surgery. The main goal of the treatment is to eliminate the infection and to secure good integration and function of the newly inserted implants. There are some protocols worked out for different courses of the infection, describing one-stage or two-stage procedures. The latter seems to be safer, especially in using non-cemented implants in revision.

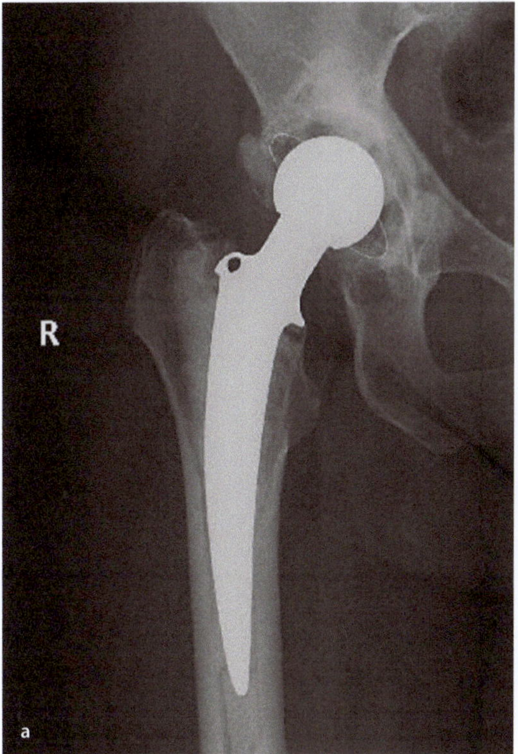

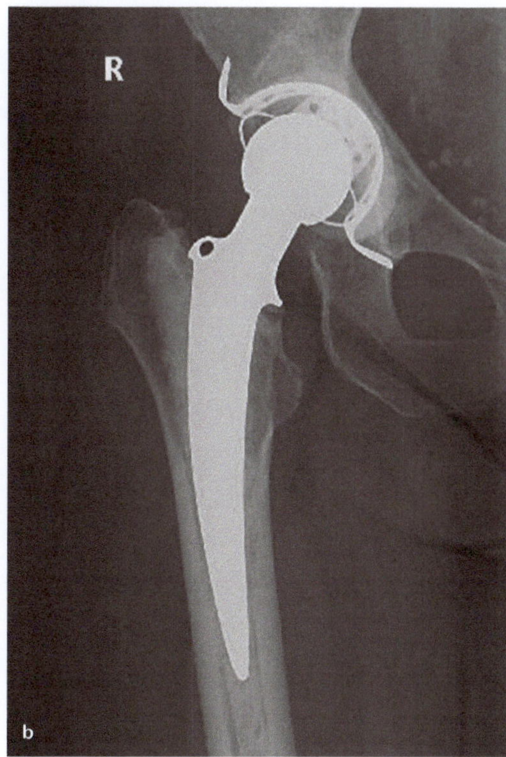

Fig. 16.5. a Loosening of the cemented cup. **b.** Cemented cup after revision with use of bone-grafting and reinforcement metallic net

References

Danish Hip Arthroplasty Register (2008) Annual Report 2007. Affiliated Center for Clinical Databases, Department of Clinical Epidemiology, Aarhus

Fink B, Grossmann A, Fuerst M, Schäfer P, Frommelt L (2009) Two-stage cementless revision of infected hip endoprostheses. Clin Orthop Relat Res 467(7): 1848–58

Götze C, Sippel C, Wendt G, Steinbeck J (2003) Limits in cementless hip revision total hip arthroplasty. Midterm experience with an oblong revision cup. Z Orthop Ihre Grenzgeb 141: 182–189

Haydon CM, Mehin R, Burnett S, Rorabeck CH, Bourne RB, McCalden RW, MacDonald SJ (2004) Revision total hip arthroplasty with use of a cemented femoral component. Results at a mean of ten years. J Bone Joint Surg Am 86-A: 1179–1185

Iorio R, Healy WL, Presutti AH (2008) A prospective outcomes analysis of femoral component fixation in revision total hip arthroplasty. J Arthroplasty 23: 662–669

Koudela K, Malotín T (2001) Reconstruction of the acetabulum during replacement of the aseptically loosened polyethylene cup. Acta Chir Orthop Traumatol Cech 68: 162–167

Kraay MJ, Goldberg VM, Fitzgerald SJ, Salata MJ (2005) Cementless two-staged total hip arthroplasty for deep periprosthetic infection. Clin Orthop Relat Res 441: 243–249

Norwegian Arthroplasty Register (2008) Annual Report 2007. Department of Orthopedic Surgery, Haukeland University, Bergen

Sanchez-Sotelo J, Berry DJ, Hanssen AD, Cabanela ME (2009) Mid-term to long-term follow-up of staged reimplantation for infected hip arthroplasty. Clin Orthop Relat Res 467: 219–224

Swedish Hip Arthroplasty Register (2007) Annual Report 2006. Sahlgrenska University Hospital, Goteborg

Templeton JE, Callaghan JJ, Goetz DD, Sullivan PM, Johnston RC (2001) Revision of a cemented acetabular component to a cementless acetabular component. A ten to fourteen-year follow-up study. J Bone Joint Surg Am 83-A: 1706–1711

Weber KL, Callaghan JJ, Goetz DD, Johnston RC (1996) Revision of a failed cemented total hip prosthesis with insertion of an acetabular component without cement and a femoral component with cement. A five to eight-year follow-up study. J Bone Joint Surg Am 78: 982–994

Yoo JJ, Kwon YS, Koo KH, Yoon KS, Kim YM, Kim HJ (2008) One-stage cementless revision arthroplasty for infected hip replacements. Int Orthop Aug 13

The Infected Implant: Revision One Stage Versus Two Stage – Introduction To Crossfire Session

Enzo Meani, Paolo Trezza

Since the beginning of human history, there has been the urge of healing, there have been the medicine men. And, quite immediately, they had to confront with the need of curing wounds, especially infected ones.

So we know from ancient cuneiform clay tablets that in the Sumerian and Assyrian-Babylonian civilization more than 4000 years ago honey was well known as a wound-dressing, as it was in Egypt and in China.[1]

In the ancient Greece, Hippocrates, by everyone named as the Father of the Medical Art (sounds much like Artz Medezin), wrote that »honey cleans sores and ulcers of the lips, heals carbuncles and running sore«.

Through the long and shining history of the Roman culture and well kept into the minds of the legions field surgeons (cerusici) the empirical use of transdermal antiseptics for the cure and the avoidance of complicated infection came to the middle age cloisters were the monks brought to perfection the study of the officinalia.

The modern antibiotic era has to be set in 1928, though, with the discovery of penicillin by sir Alexander Fleming.

As a first sentence, and step towards the discussion, it is important to say that the therapy of the bone infections is a combined surgical and medical treatment.

When evaluating the surgical treatment of an infected lower limb articular prosthesis there are different options for the surgeon: the soft-tissue debridement, the one-stage revision, the two-stage revision, the arthrodesis and at last the limb amputation (for the knee).

The soft-tissue debridement has to be chosen only when approaching an early infection, which had an onset within 3–6 weeks from the arthroplasty implantation. In any case (early or delayed clinical appearance of prosthetic infections) there is always a very early formation of the adhesive colonies forming the biofilm coating of the metal components of the prosthetic implant.

The surgical debridement and a subsequent systemic therapy are, on the other hand, effective against the planctonic colonies of the bacterial strains.

The surgical therapy for late and chronic infections has its key concept in the complete removal of the metal components of the implant.

This has to be followed by the accurate and deep debridement of the periprosthetic soft tissues.

The third moment of the therapy is the revision prosthesis implant. On this issue the authors,

---

[1] Edwin Smith Papyrus, written around 1700 BC, thought to be based on material from as early as 3000 BC. at the Rare Book Room, New York Academy of Medicine.

and the surgeons in their everyday practice, are divided between those who consider it as safe to put in place the new components during the same surgical session of the removal and those who think it as safer to use a temporary antibiotic-loaded bone-cement spacer and to put the definitive prosthesis in place in a second surgical stage. This choice will be the issue of this crossfire.

The arthrodesis (knee) or the Girdlestone procedure (hip) should be performed after the failure of previous revision surgeries or in presence of a really poor bone stock and soft-tissue coverage. The patient's bad compliance for a long-term surgery should also affect his choice.

Limb amputation represent an extreme measure that should be reserved for highly compromised patients with bad functional prognosis of the affected articulation involved.

The systemic antibiotic therapy represents a basis of the therapy of prosthetic infections in association with the surgical time.

Nevertheless, local bactericidal action in tissues with poor capillary blood supply and an unsatisfactory action of the systemic antibiotic therapy requests an in-site antibiotic delivery to protect the implant. This goal can be easily achieved by using antibiotic-loaded bone cement.

The systemic antibiotic therapy is mandatory to kill the planctonic bacteria in the articular and periostal space while the local therapy is able to avoid the adhesion of bacterial colonies on the metal side (biofilm; Neut 2008).

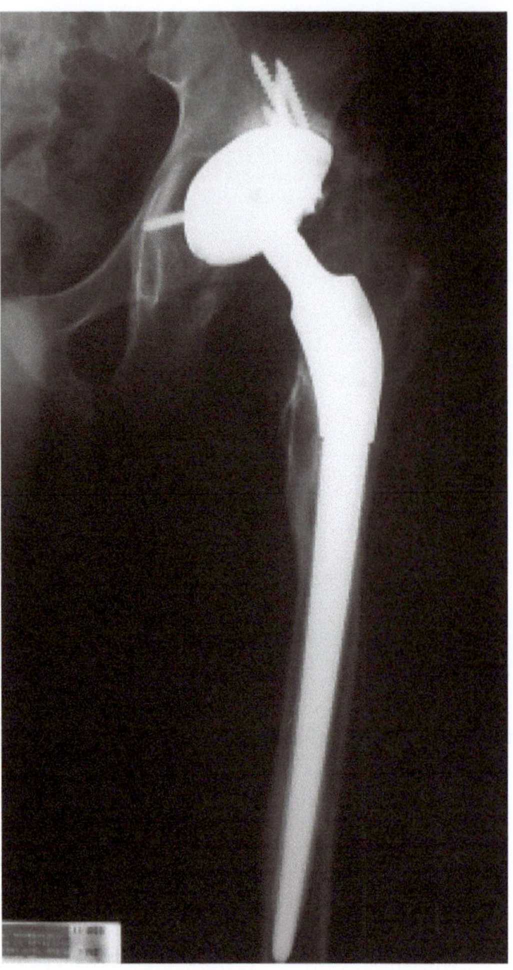

Fig. 17.1. Infected cemented primary implant prosthesis

Septic Hip Prosthesis – One-Stage Revision

One-stage surgery can be held as safe in presence of a gram-positive bacterial colonization with good periprosthetic blood supply and in absence of fistulas.

The most often isolated pathogens responsible for a prosthetic infection are gram-positive *Staphylococcus aureus* and *Staphylococcus epidermidis*, and gram-negative *Pseudomonas aeruginosa* and *Proteus*.

The radiological exclusion of osteomyelitis and the presence of a good bone stock are also key points to support this choice.

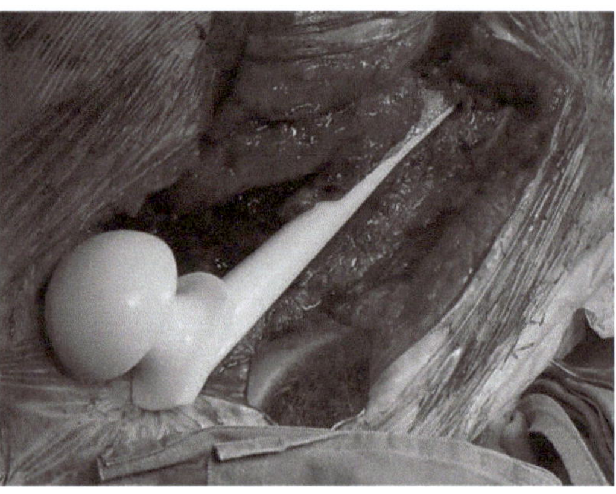

Fig. 17.2. Long-stem antibiotic-loaded bone cement to overcome the proximal femoral shaft defect after debridement

The new implant should, for the reasons said, be a cemented one and the cement should be antibiotic-loaded, at high dose, better hand-mixed on the isolated bacteria sensitivity (Hanssen and Spangehl 2004).

According to most of the literature on this topic, the recurrence of infection after one-stage surgery is about 10–23%, and in this case a new one-stage procedure should be performed (Bucholz et al. 1981; Carlsson et al. 1978; Cierney et al. 1983; Lecuire et al. 1999).

To be safe, the surgical debridement for a one-stage revision must be really radical (oncological-like) on the bone tissue, and in some cases this could bind the surgeon to use highly complex implants to overcome this demolitive approach.

Petty et al. (1978) showed the toxicity of anti-biotic-loaded cement on PMN and the concerns emerged about the long-term safe.

The use of loaded cements can be held as clinically safe also in elderly and compromised patients. The use of concentration-dependent antibiotic molecules allows a local concentration higher than the MIC but with a transient systemic concentration peak unable to cause acute renal failure (Springer et al. 2004).

Local antibiotic therapy, with the cement as a medium, can also allow a shorter systemic antibi-

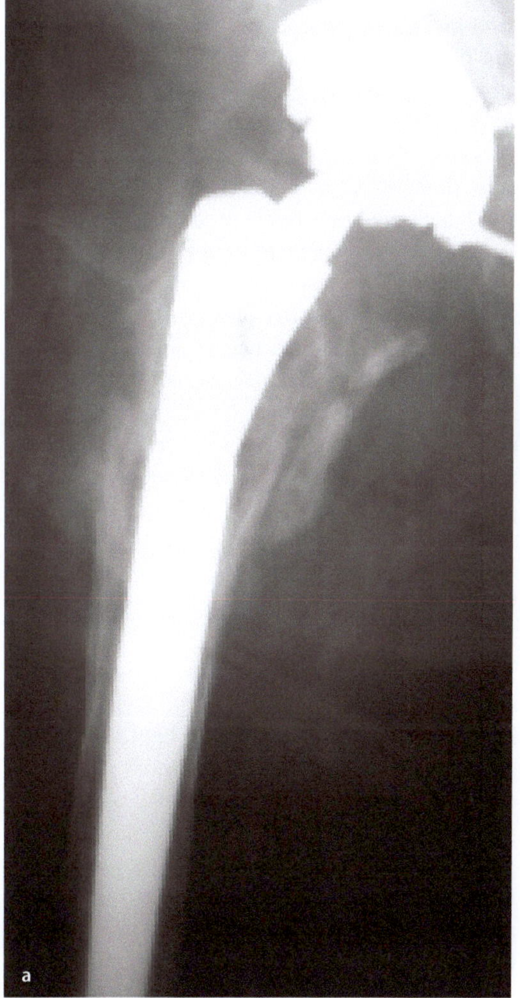

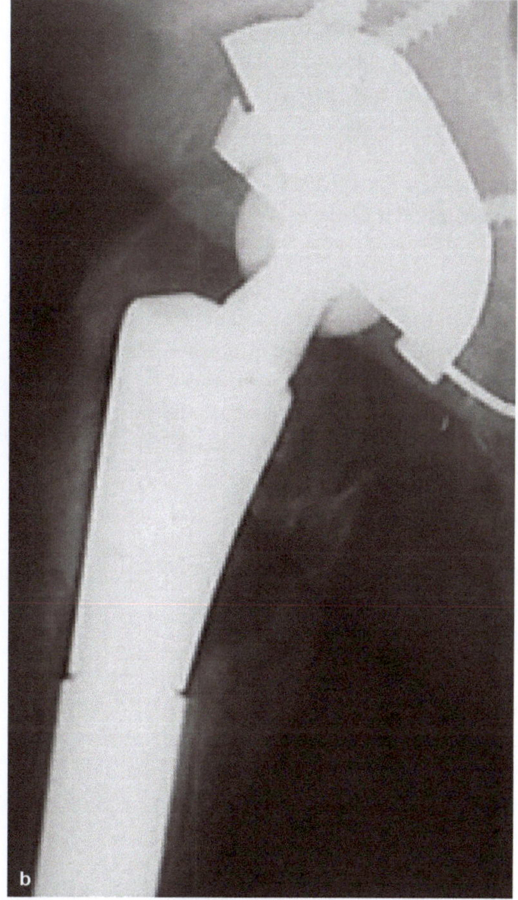

Fig. 17.3a,b. The revision prosthesis at the moment of the implantation with the use of growth factors (**a**), and after 18 months (**b**) showing a satisfactory stimulated bone growth

otic administration, reduces side effects and lowers the expenses (Stockley et al. 2008).

One of the most common issues about the use of antibiotic-loaded cement is that it will have its mechanical properties reduced, but there are studies showing that probably the shear strength would not be affected (Kilicoglu et al. 2008).

The antibiotic-loaded cement in the long period could give a positive selective pressure for small colony variants and antibiotic-resistant strains.

It should be added at least with two principles like the mix of gentamicin and clindamycin that covers almost 90% of the bacteria most often involved, answering the actual need to avoid the positive selection of small colony variants and MRSA.

For the future the addition of commercial bone cements with glycopeptides, such as vancomycin or even teicoplanin will represent the way for fighting the staphyloccocal colonization of the implants (Gallo et al. 2005).

Septic Hip Prosthesis – Two-Stage Revision: Reasons of a Choice

In the bone-cement spacer, industrial- or custom-made, we can achieve a really higher antibiotic concentration than in the thin cement layer around the metal stem in one-stage surgery.

Two surgical times allow a better debridement and a more conservative treatment (at least at the beginning) to the bone stock and this would also allow the use of non-cemented prosthesis.

Many authors report satisfactory results for this technique (Younger et al. 1997; Leunig et al. 1998; Magnan et al. 2001; Takahira et al. 2003; Evans 2004; Hsieh et al. 2005).

We think it is a reasonable choice to use pre-formed spacers because they can assure a known release of the principles (> MIC for at least 7 months) with a high local defence of the area debrided (Bertazzoni Minelli et al. 2004). They have a good mechanical resistance, if compared with custom-made ones, and long-stem models allow to overcome the femoral proximal bone loss. Furthermore, they cut the surgical time in a relevant amount.

The use of cemented prosthesis at the reimplantation has its strong points in the prolonged local release of antibiotic after time two, in it less expense, and in the easier removal as regards to a well-integrated uncemented prosthesis if a re-revision is needed.

In our unit experience, an uncemented prosthesis has to be preferred because of the doubts about fragilization of the antibiotic-loaded cement in the long-term fixation (Bucholz 1986).

There is no real need for further local antibiotic therapy at lower doses than those used in the spacer, because to be effective it should be high dose and, even better, added on the basis of the pathogen isolation on culture (Thomes et al. 2002; Hendriks et al. 2005; van de Belt et al. 2000).

Above all, there are good long-term results with non-cemented revision prosthesis in aseptic loosening and more: modularity is helpful for balancing intra-operatively legs length, offset and muscular tension, allowing a more »close to nature« and functional result (Kraay et al. 2005; Mitchell et al. 2003; Haddad et al. 2000; Fehring et al. 1999).

Distal fixation, which can be obtained with press fit stems, overcomes proximal femoral bone loss which are quite frequent after deep debridement surgery and primary implant removal.

As a last advantage, with an uncemented prosthetic system, bone graft plus growth factors like BMP-2 or BMP-7, when needed, may be securely added with no elevation of the risk of a infective relapse or bacterial growth cross-reactions (Hsieh et al. 2005). But, finally, we want to give room to the argumentations of those who respectively support one-stage and two-stage revision technique.

Conclusions

There are still many controversies about the one-stage or two-stages protocol in the revision of an infected prosthetic implant. The fight against infections is as old as the human history. Today the orthopaedic surgeons have often to deal with the prosthetic infection and with the requirement to perform a safe and durable revision surgery of the implants. If there is an overall consensus on the need to remove all the infected metal components, the authors and the surgeons in their practice are divided about the experience of re-implanting the new prosthesis during the same surgical time whether doing it in a second surgical time to eradicate the infection. In this case it is mandatory to implant a temporary bone-cement spacer loaded with antibiotics to avoid shortening of the limb and to maintain locally the drug level above the MIC. Our assignment here is to introduce the different opinions from those who support one-stage revision surgery and those who think two stages are safer.

References

Bertazzoni Minelli E, Benini A, Magnan B, Bartolozzi P (2004) Release of gentamicin and vancomycin from temporary human hip spacers in two-stage revision of infected arthroplasty. J Antimicrob Chemother 53: 329–334

Buchholz HW, Elson RA, Engelbrecht E, Lodenkämper H, Röttger J, Siegel A (1981) Management of deep infection of total hip replacement. J Bone Joint Surg Br 63-B: 342–353

Buchholz HW (1986) Megaprosthesis and infection after total hip prosthesis. Acta Orthop Belg 52: 360–367

Carlsson AS, Josefsson G, Lindberg L (1978) Revision with gentamicin-impregnated cement for deep infections in total hip arthroplasties. J Bone Joint Surg Am 60: 1059–1064

Cierny G, DiPasquale D (2002) Periprosthetic total joint infections: staging, treatment, and outcomes. Clin Orthop Relat Res 403: 23–28

Evans RP (2004) Successful treatment of total hip and knee infection with articulating antibiotic components: a modified treatment method. Clin Orthop Relat Res 427: 37–46

Fehring TK, Calton TF, Griffin WL (1999) Cementless fixation in 2-stage reimplantation for periprosthetic sepsis. J Arthroplasty 14: 175–181

Gallo J, Kolár M, Florschütz AV, Novotný R, Pantcek R, Kesselová M (2005) In vitro testing of gentamicin-vancomycin loaded bone cement to prevent prosthetic joint infection. Biomed Pap Med Fac Univ Palacky Olomouc Czech Repub 149: 153–158

Haddad FS, Muirhead-Allwood SK, Manktelow AR, Bacarese-Hamilton I (2000) Two-stage uncemented revision hip arthroplasty for infection. J Bone Joint Surg Br 82: 689–694

Hanssen AD, Spangehl MJ (2004) Practical applications of antibiotic-loaded bone cement for treatment of infected joint replacements. Clin Orthop Relat Res 427: 79–85

Hendriks JG, Neut D, van Horn JR, van der Mei HC, Busscher HJ (2005) Bacterial survival in the interfacial gap in gentamicin-loaded acrylic bone cements. J Bone Joint Surg Br 87: 272–276

Hsieh PH et al. (2005) Treatment of deep infection of the hip associated with massive bone loss: two-stage revision with an antibiotic-loaded interim cement prosthesis followed by reconstruction with allograft. J Bone Joint Surg Br 87: 770–775

Kilicoglu O, Koyuncu LO, Ozden VE, Bozdag E, Sunbuloglu E, Yazicioglu O (2008) Effect of antibiotic loading on the shear strength at the stem-cement interface (Shear strength of antibiotic loaded cement). Int Orthop 32: 437–441

Kraay MJ, Goldberg VM, Fitzgerald SJ, Salata MJ (2005) Cementless two-staged total hip arthroplasty for deep periprosthetic infection. Clin Orthop Relat Res 441: 243–249

Lecuire F, Collodel M, Basso M, Rubini J, Gontier D, Carrère J (1999) Revision of infected total hip prostheses by ablation reimplantation of an uncemented prosthesis. 57 case reports. Rev Chir Orthop Reparatrice Appar Mot 85: 337–348

Leunig M, Chosa E, Speck M, Ganz R (1998) A cement spacer for two-stage revision of infected implants of the hip joint. Int Orthop 22: 209–214

Magnan B, Regis D, Biscaglia R, Bartolozzi P (2001) Preformed acrylic bone cement spacer loaded with antibiotics: use of two-stage procedure in 10 patients because of infected hips after total replacement. Acta Orthop Scand 72: 591–594

Meani E, Romanò CL, Crosby L, Hofman G (2007) Infections and local therapy in orthopedic surgery. Springer, Berlin Heidelberg New York Tokyo

Mitchell PA, Masri BA, Garbuz DS, Greidanus NV, Duncan CP (2003) Cementless revision for infection following total hip arthroplasty. Instr Course Lect 52: 323-330

Neut D (2008 Pros and cons of antibiotic-loaded bone cement. Lecture at the XXVII° annual Meeting of the EBJIS, Barcelona, 18–20 September 2008

Petty W (1978) The effect of methylmetacrylate on bacterial phagocytosis and killing by human polymorphonuclear leukocytes. J Bone Joint Surg Am 60: 752–757

Springer BD, Lee GC, Osmon D, Haidukewych GJ, Hanssen AD, Jacofsky DJ (2004) Systemic safety of high-dose antibiotic-loaded cement spacers after resection of an infected total knee arthroplasty. Clin Orthop Relat Res 427: 47–51

Stockley I, Mockford BJ, Hoad-Reddick A, Norman P (2008) The use of two-stage exchange arthroplasty with depot antibiotics in the absence of long-term antibiotic therapy in infected total hip replacement. J Bone Joint Surg Br 90: 145–148

Takahira N, Itoman M, Higashi K, Uchiyama K, Miyabe M, Naruse K (2003) Treatment outcome of two-stage revision total hip arthroplasty for infected hip arthroplasty using antibiotic-impregnated cement spacer. J Orthop Sci 8: 26–31

Thomes B, Murray P, Bouchier-Hayes D (2002) Development of resistant strains of Staphylococcus epidermidis on gentamicin-loaded bone cement in vivo. J Bone Joint Surg Br 84: 758–760

van de Belt H, Neut D, Schenk W, van Horn JR, van der Mei HC, Busscher HJ (2000) Gentamicin release from polymethylmethacrylate bone cements and Staphylococcus aureus biofilm formation. Acta Orthop Scand 71: 625–629

Younger AS, Duncan CP, Masri BA, McGraw RW (1997) The outcome of two-stage arthroplasty using a custom-made interval spacer to treat the infected hip. J Arthroplasty 12: 615–623

One Stage Revision – Favourite Option?

Götz von Foerster, Lars Frommelt

Introduction

Periprosthetic infection of total joint replacement is a rare complication of procedure frequently performed. Due to the fact that periprosthetic infection is a foreign-body-associated infection established in bone tissue, this infection is difficult to treat. Antimicrobial agents alone fail to control this disease. As in other foreign-body-associated infections, surgical intervention is necessary together with antibiotic therapy. Except for early not established infection surgical removal of foreign material must be done for the control of these lesions.

Additional to surgery antibiotic therapy it is useful to ensure the success of this procedure. There are two ways of administering antimicrobial agents by systemically administration or locally fixed to a delivery vehicle. Most common is the incorporation in polymethylmetacrylate (PMMA) bone cement as introduced by Buchholz and Engelbrecht (1970). Antibiotic-loaded bone cement (ALAC) is essential in one-stage revision and useful in multiple-stage revision if spacers are used (Robbins et al. 2001). Whereas in recommendations from US-American authors (Hanssen and Spangehl 2004) the empirical choice in high concentration is preferred, the authors use targeted antimicrobial agents against the causative patho-gen in one-stage revision of periprosthetic infection. In the ENDO-Klinik in Hamburg meanwhile over 7000 one-stage revisions are performed with good success (Buchholz et al. 1981; von Foerster et al. 1991). The intention of this article is to demonstrate the technique used and to point out the prerequisites necessary for one-staged exchange revision in periprosthetic infection (Fig. 18.1).

Method of One-Staged Revision

One-stage revision is based upon knowledge of the pathogen, radical surgery including removal of all foreign material at site of infection and meticulous performed débridement of bone and soft tissue, cleansing of the bone tissue by pulsating jet lavage, implantation of total joint replacement using PMMA bone cement with antimicrobial agents incorporated according to the susceptibility of the pathogen, and short term systemic antibiotic therapy for about two weeks.

Prerequisites for One-Staged Revision

One-staged revision requires preoperative investigation of the pathogen, bone stock that allows implantation of another total joint replacement,

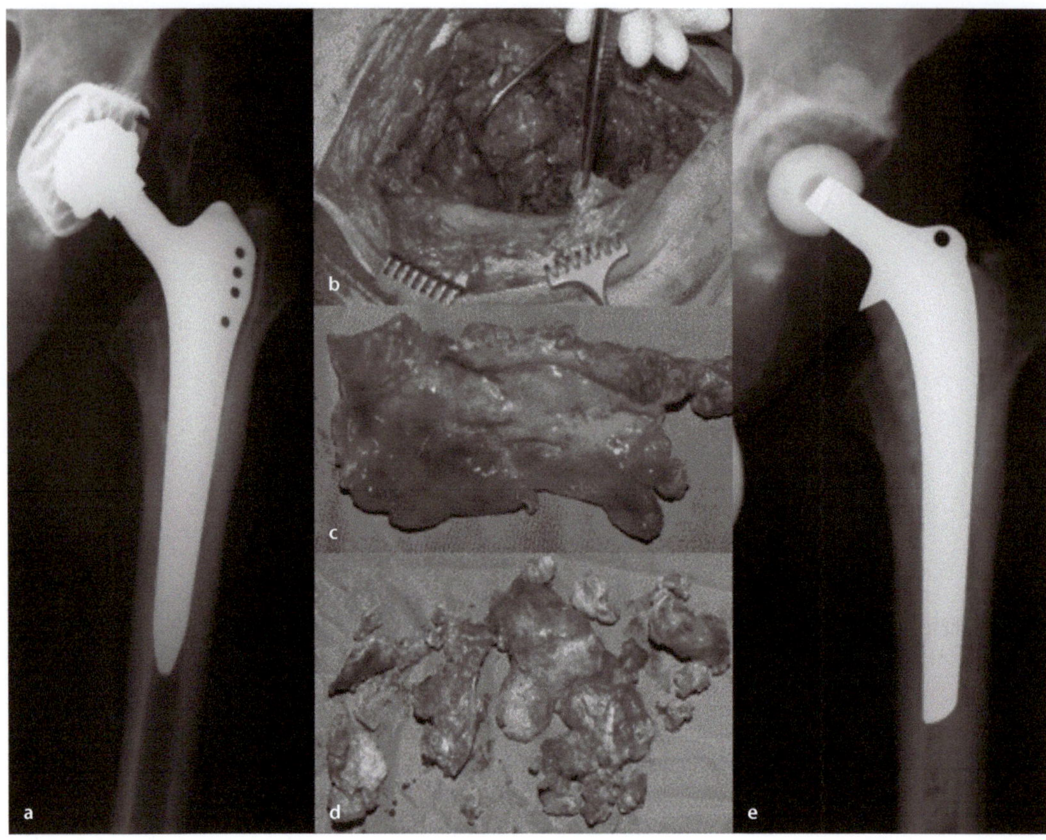

Fig. 18.1. a Preoperative X-ray, **b** intraoperative: start of debridement of the infectious membrane, **c** intraoperative: greater part of the infective membrane, **d** intraoperative: resected tissue due to infection (debridement), **e** postoperative X-ray

and effective antibiotic available for application to PMMA bone cement without harm for the patient.

Diagnostic of the Pathogen

In case of empyema or if fistula is present it is easy to ensure periprosthetic infection. Unfortunately, a lot of these infections show only few symptoms leading to the diagnosis of infection. In low-grade infection often pain in most cases combined with slight elevation of C-reactive protein (CRP) are the only and often misleading signs of illness. These conditions have to be suspected as periprosthetic infection until proven from other origin (Fink et al. 2008; Frommelt 2008).

Under these conditions the detection cytology of the synovial fluid is of worth to answer the question whether infection is present. This can be done by semi-quantitative count in the smears or better, as proposed by Trampuz et al. (2004), mechanical count and differentiation of the white blood cells in synovial fluid by blood-cell analyzer. Cell count above 1700/µL in presence of artificial knee replacement and presence of more than 65% of neutrophils give strong suggestion that infectious disease is present. This will be proven by detection of the pathogen.

Detection of the pathogen has to respect the special condition of bacteria causing foreign-body-associated infection. The specimen must be representative for the site of infection and because bacteria low in number and altered in contrast to vial planktonic ones it is necessary to breed cultures for at least 14 days and to use highly enriched media to recover these germs (Schäfer et al. 2008). Crucial for detection is that the clinical microbiologist is familiar with this problem and gets the information that a foreign-body infection is suspected.

Choice of Antimicrobial Agents

Antimicrobial agents chosen for admixing to PMMA bone cement must be able to be eluted from bone cement, resist heat resulting from polymerization of PMMA, must be effective in the bacterial pathogen, and must not result in adverse effects like allergy in the patient. These antibiotics must be available as powder. Whenever possible admixing by hand in the theatre should be avoided and industrial preparations have to be used if available.

In case of one-stage revision empirical therapy is inappropriate. Specific antibiotic therapy according to the individual pathogen's susceptibility pattern has to be performed.

The same applies to perioperative systemic antimicrobial therapy that have to respect the pharmacokinetic and pharmacodynamic properties of the antibiotic agents.

Patient's Condition

The patient must be able to undergo the procedure with reasonable risk assessment. No adverse effects or risks including allergic reaction for antimicrobial agents used must be detected in the patients history or be likely from metabolic condition of the patient.

Quality of bone stock must allow direct re-implantation of total joint replacement (TJR) within the same procedure.

Surgeon and the Team Behind

For periprosthetic infection especially in low-grade infection needs not only an experienced and well-skilled surgeon but also a team of different medical specialties in order to manage problems in diagnostics and to optimize the outcome for the patient.

For the diagnostic period the communication between the surgeon and the clinical microbiologist enables the laboratory to optimize the recovery of pathogens in this infection and give appropriate advice for clinical use of antibiotics needed. Optimal imaging of the site of infection enables the surgeon to choose a prosthetic device adequate for the anatomical condition in the individual case including e.g. custom-made devises. In elderly patients anaesthesia is of outstanding impact in order to minimize possible complication. Directly after the patient recovers from the procedure, physical therapy has to start to give optimal motility back to the patient. In septic revision this is of special interest because radical debridement may cause functional defects, which have to be compensated.

Technique of One-Staged Revision Including Pre-Operative Precautions and Postoperative Nursery

The surgical technique of one-staged revision and precautions pre- and postoperatively required are demonstrated by case reports.

Case Report 1

A 68-years old female patient was operated on for osteoarthritis of the left hip ten months ago and uncemented artificial hip replacement was implanted. During the postoperative period no abnormalities were recorded. Unspecific complaints increasing over the time occurred in the following period. About 4 weeks before consulting the surgeon, the patient reported starting weight-bearing-dependent pain of increasing strength. Meanwhile she is limited in walking short distances.

Inspection shows no signs of local infection as redness, swelling, or hyperthermia. Condition of the scar is bland. Medical examination demonstrates slight pain in rotation and less in compression, no signs of loosening of the THR (total hip replacement).

X-ray of the left hip shows a well-implanted cementless THR in regular position. No signs of loosening are reported.

Laboratory tests demonstrate only a slight anaemia and C-reactive protein is elevated up to 22 mg/L (reference: < 5 mg/L).

Because low-grade infection was suspected, an aspiration of joint fluid was performed. About 5 mL slightly cloudy synovial fluids were obtained. Cell count resulted in 2200 cells/µL and 75% neutrophils. After 8 days of breeding culture media shows growth of *Staphylococcus epidermidis* in microbiological investigation.

One-stage revision was planned in order to replace the uncemented THR by a cemented THR using specific ALAC for fixation. The choice of antimicrobial agents was done according to susceptibility testing of the pathogen for admixture to PMMA bone cement and systemic therapy as well: 1 g clindamycin and 1 g gentamicin for local therapy in bone cement and flucloxacillin intravenously (4 times 2 g/IV/day) for 14 days.

Preoperatively no antibiotics were administered.

After incision of the skin, subcutaneous tissue appeared to be free of infection. The fascia was exposed and after incision the tissue underneath looked slightly suspicious for infection. Subsequently, the M. piriformis was dissected and the tendon was cut nearby the insertion at the femur. Dorsal incision of the capsular of the joint was done. At the moment of incision cloudy fluid evacuates form the joint's inner compartment. Proceeding further and after luxation of the femoral component typical inflammatory signs are found throughout the synovialis with redness and proliferation. After exposition of the shaft, infected tissue appears starting at the connection between femur and prosthesis while the shaft was not loosened clinically. After disconnection of the artificial femoral head an extractor is mounted and following loosening the bony interface by special chisels the shaft can be extracted without inducing femoral fracture. Specimens for microbiologic investigation are taken from the synovialis and bone tissue from the inner part of the femur proximal and distal as well.

Next, the well-incorporated cup is exposed and slackened by using chisels directly along the rim of the cup whereas some space must be formed in the lower caudal region in order to ease the extraction of the cup. After removal of the cup specimen for bacteriological examination are obtained by curettage of acetabular area.

After removal of the THR and sampling for microbiological examination systemic antimicrobial therapy is started.

Debridement of bone and soft tissue is performed until apparently uninfected tissue is reached. Synovialis and capsular tissue is removed. The whole frontier to uninfected tissue is groped around for residual niches or small abscesses in the soft tissue. Next the cleansing and cutting of bone tissue is performed. Subsequently, the total situs is exposed to pulsating jet lavage and finally Lavasept, an antiseptic solution, is administered into the area of revision and exposed during 8 min to the antiseptic.

Re-implantation of THR starts with the application of ALAC in the acetabulum and insertion of the cup. After the bone cement has been cured, a test reposition is done using a dummy prosthesis for the shaft in order to define the length to prevent future luxation. Then the dummy prosthesis is removed and the bone bed rinsed again prior to application of ALAC, insertion of the definite shaft, adaptation of the head to the conus, and definite reposition of THR is done.

Drainage tubes are put into position. If possible, refixation of the M. piriformis is done. Next the fascia is adapted and closed »leak-proven«. The subcutaneous drainage is put into position and sutures are used to stabilize subcutaneous tissue and to close the wound. After draping with elastic bandages of the whole limb, X-ray is performed for documentation.

Drainages are removed on the second day after operation and physical therapy starts with moderate exercises and mobilization.

For monitoring of healing and control of infection the wound is inspected every day and especially laboratory tests for CRP are performed. If CRP declines to the reference range or beneath the preoperative value this is a good prognostic sign as to the control of infection.

In the demonstrated case regular wound-healing took place and CRP came down in time. From 3 out of 4 intraoperative obtained biopsies *Staphylococcus epidermidis* were recovered showing the identical susceptibility pattern as compared with the strain preoperatively found. Systemic antibiotic therapy with flucloxacillin was continued for 14 days after revision. Subsequently, the patient was transferred to a rehabilitation unit.

No recurrence of infection was found in the follow-up 2 years later. Range of motion and mobility were fair, CRP was not elevated and the X-ray showed a regular anatomical position of the THR without signs of loosening.

Case Report 2

An 84-years old male suffered from periprosthetic infection of the right hip. A cemented THR was implanted 7 years before. The patient underwent transurethral resection of the prostate 3 months before. Postoperatively, urinary tract infection occurred and was cured by oral antibiotic therapy with chinolones. Shortly after this episode he developed slight but increasing pain in the right hip. He went to see the orthopaedic surgeon because of pain, swelling and redness in the area of the right hip.

Aspiration of joint fluid was done. Synovial fluid showed 2500 cells/µL and 70% of neutrophils. In microbiological investigation *Pseudomonas aeruginosa* was detected after 6 days of incubation.

One-staged revision was performed. When cement was removed, part of the distal cement got lost in the depth of the femur (Fig. 18.2) and was left there because it seemed impossible to remove with reasonable effort.

Postoperatively, the patient recovered in time, wound-healing showed no complication, CRP normalized in time, and the patient was transferred to the rehabilitation unit in time.

Six months later recurrence of pain was reported to increase over the time. Medical examination showed no signs of inflammation locally but CRP was slightly elevated again. Microbiological investigation of joint fluid showed growth of *Pseudomonas aeruginosa* again. Because persisting infection was considered another one-staged revision was performed. Intraoperatively signs of infection were found especially in the area of the bone cement left at the time of revision before.

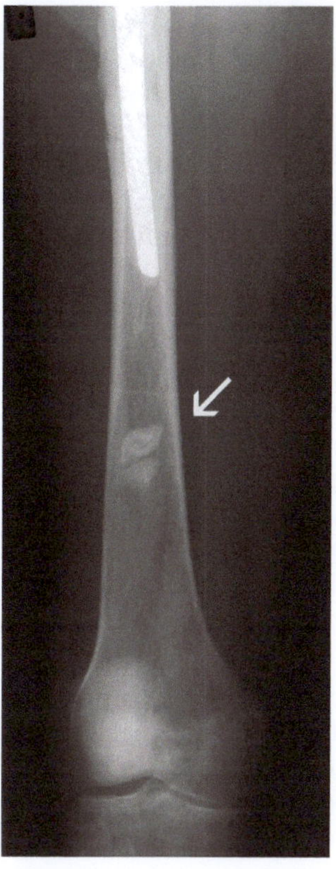

 Fig. 18.2. Bone cement lost in removal (flash): Bone cement must be removed even if removal is difficult because of the localization

Impact of Debridement and Removal of Bone Cement

As therapy of periprosthetic infection is surgical removal of infected bone tissue and soft tissue involved. Debridement has to be performed meticulously and radically. Elements of debridement are excision of sinuses, drainage of all abscesses including hidden ones in anatomical niches and removal of all foreign material, membranes, cement, plugs and any potentially infected soft tissue.

Especially removal of bone cement may be difficult. For extraction of bone cement suitable instruments as osteotomes and chisels in various size and thickness must be available. Furthermore, instruments for curettage, ball-headed reamers and self-cutting cement extractors, are necessary.

Before removal of the prosthesis, bone cement in the area of the Trochanter major has to be removed as far as possible in order to prevent femoral fracture while extracting the femoral stem of the prosthesis. The remaining cement mantel has to be removed step by step. Within the first 5–7 cm bone cement can be broken into small pieces using chisels which can easily be extracted. For thin parts of the mantel ball-headed reamers may be of advantage.

In deeper areas with solid bone-cement plaque self-cutting extractors are of benefit. Bone-cement pieces measuring approximately 2 cm should be extracted carefully. Beyond the femoral isthmus the method cannot be used for preventing femoral fracture. Here fenestration of cortical bone distal to the isthmus may be necessary to remove bone cement.

In highly curved stems and in extremely long prosthesis extraction of bone cement from the distal part of the femur is not possible. In these cases fenestration, sometimes double fenestration, of cortical bone is inevitable to remove all parts of cement. Fenestration if necessary should be performed from ventral exposure.

The necessity to remove bone cement completely contradicts the cement-in-cement technique, as it is of advantage in aseptic revision. This technique is inadequate in periprosthetic infection and leads to persisting infection.

Antimicrobial Agents in One-Staged Revision

For one-staged revision the antibiotics administered locally are imperatively necessary. Widely use for administering antimicrobial agents acrylic bone cement is used even though other carriers like bone grafts are used for this purpose (Winkler et al. 2008).

Antibiotics admixed to bone cement must be heat-stable and delivery from cured bone cement must be proven in experiments. Antibiotics can be used only as powder, and this has to be mixed carefully with the polymer powder of PMMA bone cement. Whenever available, industrial preparations should be used because they are superior to any hand-made preparation with respect to elution properties and stability of the bone cement. Unfortunately, many antibiotics necessary to control periprosthetic infection are not available in such preparations.

In addition to local antibiotics systemically administered antibiotic therapy starts for 14 days after samples for microbiological investigation are drawn during revision.

The combination of local antibiotics allows systemic antibiotic therapy for only a short period.

Advantages of One-Staged Revision

In one-staged revision only one operation is performed in most of the patient. That means the risk of revision-associated perioperative complications is reduced for those patients, which have not to undergo another revision.

The combination of locally administered antibiotics allows reducing the period of systemic antibiotics to 10–24 days in case of uncomplicated postoperative healing.

If any doubt occurs during procedure, the tactic can be switched to two-staged revision without any problems. The prerequisites are sufficient for this surgical attempt as well.

For more than 80% of the patients no further surgery is necessary (Langlais et al. 2003).

Limits of One-Staged Revision

One-staged revision is not possible if no antimicrobial agents are applicable because of the resistance pattern of the causing bacterial pathogen, allergy in the patient, or if suitable antibiotics are not eluted from PMMA bone cement.

One-staged revision is inadequate if no pathogen can be identified prior to revision.

If loss of bone stock or other anatomical condition does not allow the immediate re-implantation of total joint replacement, one-staged revision is not possible.

If uncemented re-implantation of total joint replacement is intended, one-staged revision is not appropriate if revision using antibiotic impregnated bone grafts is not considered.

Virulence of the pathogen or presence of sinuses is no obstacles in the experience of the authors but the surgeon must be familiar with the principles of surgery of bone infections.

Discussion

One-staged revision is an approach to periprosthetic infection that is attractive because only one procedure is necessary to control infection. Prerequisites for one-staged revision have to be respected and targeted antimicrobial therapy is imperatively necessary in this procedure.

Compared with two- or multi-staged revision most of the elements of treatment are identical or at least comparable. In both approaches diagnosis of infection and detection of the bacterial pathogen must be undertaken prior to revision. If the detection of the pathogens fails, one-stage revision is not possible. Two- or multiple-staged revision is possible but only empirical antimicrobial therapy is possible, which is in so far of disadvantage as the susceptibility pattern of bacteria is varying to an extend that is hardly to predict.

As to the surgical procedure itself with respect to debridement and radical removal of foreign material there is no difference in both approaches.

At present re-implantation of uncemented prosthesis requires two-stage revision because the possibility of sufficient local application of antibiotics is not established now.

Most advantages apply to the patient himself. For the patient the infection can be controlled in more than 80% with only one revision. For the failures in the first revision another surgical intervention gives a fair chance to solve the problem. This is not only of comfort for the patient but in elderly patients with high co-morbidity a one-staged procedure is an approach that reduces the risk of perioperative complications by performing only one revision in most of them.

Both methods need an experienced surgeon who is familiar with surgery of bone infection apart from intervention surgery in life-threatening

septicemia where removal of the foreign material may be life-saving.

The history in the ENDO-Klinik in Hamburg shows that in the result for control of infection raised from 75% to meanwhile more than 85%. That means one-staged revision requires, as well as other methods, a learning curve. By instruction and surveillance of surgeons in training by experienced instructors this learning curve can be cut down to a certain extent. This applies to two-staged revision as well and leads to the authors' opinion that these revisions whether one- ore more staged should be performed in specialized centers. Centers like this additionally provide the surgeon with the diagnostic facilities necessary and give the possibility of cooperation with other experienced medical specialists. Of outstanding impact is the cooperation with a clinical microbiologist or an infectious-disease specialist.

Conclusion

One-staged revision is an option in the therapy of periprosthetic infection that consists from identical or minimum similar prerequisites as two- or multiple-staged revision.

Crucial for success in the control of infection is the knowledge of the causative pathogen prior to revision. Another essential element is targeted administering of antibiotics locally admixed with PMMA bone cement together with systemic antibiotic therapy.

Of special impact is the debridement and meticulously performed removal of all foreign material, which should be done by a surgeon experienced in the surgery of bone infections.

One-staged as well as two-staged revisions should be performed in specialized centers where facilities for optimal diagnostics are available and a cooperation with other medical specialists is possible.

The patient's benefit is lowering the risk of perioperative complications by performing only one revision in most of the cases.

One-staged revision is not suitable for interventional surgery in life threatening disease like septicemia caused by periprosthetic infection.

Advantages of One-Stage Revision

- One procedure in most cases (80–90%)
- One stay in hospital
- Only risk of complication in one procedure
- Possibility to switch into a two-stage procedure (if any problem occurs)

References

Buchholz HW, Elson RA, Engelbrecht E, Lodenkämper H, Rötger J, Siegel A (1981) Management of deep infection of total hip replacement. J Bone Joint Surg Br 63-B: 342–353

Buchholz HW, Engelbracht H (1970) Über die Depotwirkung einiger Antibiotika mit dem Kunstharz Palacos. Chirurg 41: 511–515

Fink B, Makowiak C, Fuerst M, Berger I, Schäfer P, Frommelt L (2008) The value of synovial biopsy, joint aspiration and C-reactive protein in the diagnosis of late peri-prosthetic infection of total knee replacement. J Bone Joint Surg Br 90: 874–878

Frommelt L (2008) Gelenkpunktat und Erregernachweis bei periprothetischer Infektion. Orthopäde 37: 1027–1036

Hanssen AD, Spangehl MJ (2004) Practical application of antibiotic loaded bone cement for treatment of infected joint replacement. Clin Orthop Relat Res 427: 79–85

Langlais F, Lambotte JC, Thomazeau (2003) Treatment of infected total hip replacement. Eur Instruc Course Lect EFFORT 6: 158–167

Robbins GM, Masri BA, Grabuz DS, Ducan CP (2001) Primary total hip arthroplasty after infection. J Bone Joint Surg 83-A: 601–617

Schäfer P, Fink B, Sandow D, Margul A, Berger I, Frommelt L (2008) Prolonged bacterial culture to identify late periprosthetic joint infection: a promising strategy. 471: 1403–1409

Trampuz A, Hanssen AD, Osmon DR, Mandrekar J, Steckelberg JM, Patel (2004) Synovial fluid leukocyte count and differential for the diagnosis of prosthetic knee infection. Am J Med 117: 556–562

Von Foerster G. Klüber D, Käbler U (1991) Mittel- und langfristige Ergebnisse nach Behandlung von 118 periprothetischen Infektionen nach Kniegelenksersatz durch einzeitige Austauschoperation. Orthopäde 20: 244–252

Winkler H, Stoiber A, Kaudela K, Winter F, Mentschik F (2008) One stage uncemented revision of infected total hip replacement using cancellous allgraft bone impregnated with antibiotics. J Bone Joint Surg Br 90-B: 1580–1584

Advantages of Two-Stage Revision Arthroplasty

Filippo Randelli, Alberto Aliprandi, Lorenzo Banci, Luca Sconfienza, Francesco Sardanelli

Background

Infection after total hip arthroplasty is an orthopaedic surgeon major concern. Overall infection incidence has not been reduced in the last few decades (Charnley 1972) assessing its incidence between 0.5% and 2% for primary total hip replacement and around 4% for partial hip arthroplasty (Wilson et al. 2008) and for revision. Diagnosis and treatment are often long and difficult and final results unpredictable.

Prevention is a key issue often underestimated. Patient selection and recognition of high-risk procedure for infection is the starting point (Bongartz et al. 2008). Laminar Airflow Systems popularized by John Charnley (1972; Fitzgerald et al. 1979) and the new ultraviolet light in the operating theatre (Ritter et al. 2007) seem to better reduce contamination.

Methicillin-resistant Staphylococcus aureus (MRSA; Ridgeway et al. 2005) and methicillin-resistant Staphylococcus epidermidis (MRSE) are growing everywhere, vancomycin-resistant Staphylococcus aureus (VRSA) and vancomycin-resistant Enterococci (VRE) have done their first appearance.

On the other hand, very slow growing pathogens make diagnosis very difficult and sometimes late only after a false aspetic loosening revision. In fact, it is not rare to find positive intraoperative cultures with coagulase-negative Staphylococci and Propionibacterium acnes (Marculescu et al. 2005). These bacteria grow very slow and, if not searched for, with a long period of culture and specific methods, can be undetected. Aspiration of a presumed infected hip joint can be easily falsely negative and repeated aspirations are needed in more difficult cases (Barrack et al. 1993).

The biofilm theory applied to orthopaedic implants and exposed by Gristina and Costerton in 1984 (Gristina et al. 1991) highlighted the pathogenetic basis of prosthetic implant infection in human body. Different types of bacteria grow over implant surfaces in a shield matrix, the biofilm, that protect them from immunological response and antibiotic effects. Only bacteria in the planktonic phase (out of the biofilm shield) can be easily reached and killed. Bacteria inside the biofilm are very difficult to kill and a 1000 time higher antibiotic level is needed. Furthermore, biofilm bacteria are difficult to grow in normal cultures. Thus, joint aspiration can be negative in biofilm joint infection. A way to try to isolate biofilm bacteria is a brief ultrasonication of the removed implant before culture (Nguyen et al. 2002). Because of this lack of sensitivity of established microbiological methods, molecular methods [e.g., polymerase chain reaction (PCR) and fluorescence in-situ hybridization (FISH)] seem to be more suitable for biofilm-infection detection (McDowell and Patrick 2005). Molecular methods are expensive and limited and so only patients with high suspicion of deep implant infection and repetitive negative aspiration cultures should be examined.

The suspicion of a low grade implant deep infection is made by the presence, without any other explanation, of one or the combination of loosening, pain, elevation of ESR, CRP (Bottner and Sculco 2001) and recently interleukine-6 (IL-6; Bottner et al. 2007; Di Cesare et al. 2005), positive ultrasound and MRI (Johnston et al. 2007) for excessive periprosthetic fluid, positive radionuclide imaging (Reinartz et al. 2005) and more 25–50 10^9 leukocytes per liter (with neutrophil more than 80%) at aspiration (Spangehl et al. 1999).

Positron emission tomography (PET) has a very good sensitivity on localization of soft-tissue involvement in our experience (◘ Fig. 19.1).

MRI has been used recently in our institution for deep-infection diagnosis. Between May and October 2008, four patients with recently implanted hip prosthesis (four males, age range 53–78 years), who referred for symptoms and/or blood tests related to a possible prosthesis infection, underwent a MR scan of the implant. Examinations were conducted by a 1.5T-MR scan (Sonata Maestro Class, Siemens, Erlangen, Germany) and a body-flexible coil wrapping the joint.

Hip prostheses are characterized by a reduced magnetic susceptibility that produce an artefact limited to coxofemoral and proximal endodiaphiseal region. The metallic matter of the prosthesis produces a hypointense signal in all sequences, surrounded by a thin hyperintense artefact that reaches the visible cortical interface. This artefact does not allow to assess the periprosthetic bone in detail. On the other hand, soft tissues are minimally interested by the abovementioned artefacts and are therefore easily evaluable. Thanks to MR imaging features, fluid collections are easily described according to their dimensions (on three spatial planes), margins and approximate volume. Furthermore, we are able to make reliable hypothesis on the nature of the fluid contained in the collection, according to the signal obtained in different sequences. This allows to characterize a serous, haematic, purulent collection, or even an

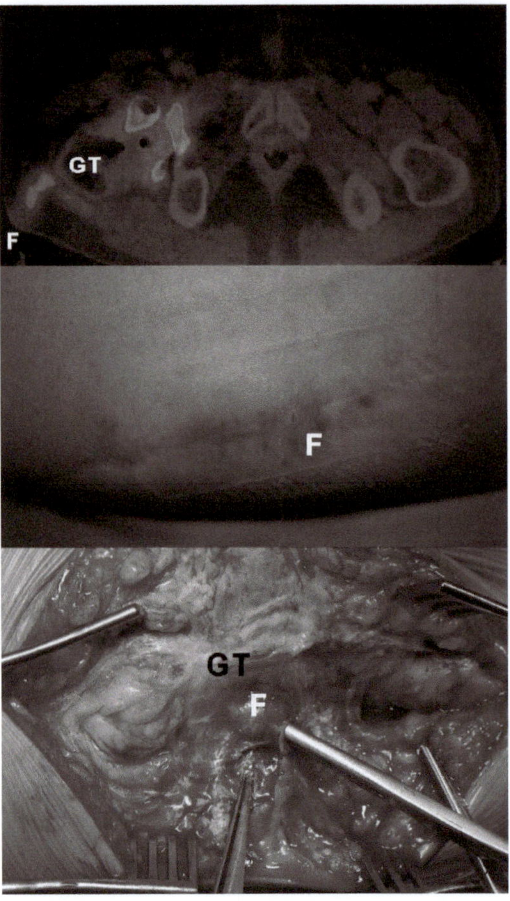

◘ **Fig. 19.1.** Positron emission tomography (PET), scar fistula (*F*) and intra-operative image of a 57-year old man with an infected right total hip replacement. Note the exact localization of soft-tissue involvement representation in PET scan. The fistula (*F*) runs from the joint space, posterior to the greater trochanter (*GT*) to reach the skin

active bleeding. Three of four patients with excessive periprosthetic fluid resulted positive at joint aspiration cultures for bacterial growth. The last patient developed purulent secretion without a positive culture (◘ Fig. 19.2).

To reach the evidence, and not only the suspicious, of a real deep infection, a positive culture or a positive molecular method should be present. Histological analysis for predicting the presence of microorganisms at the time of reimplantation has been described as usefulness. In fact, the probability of infection is high when at least five neu-

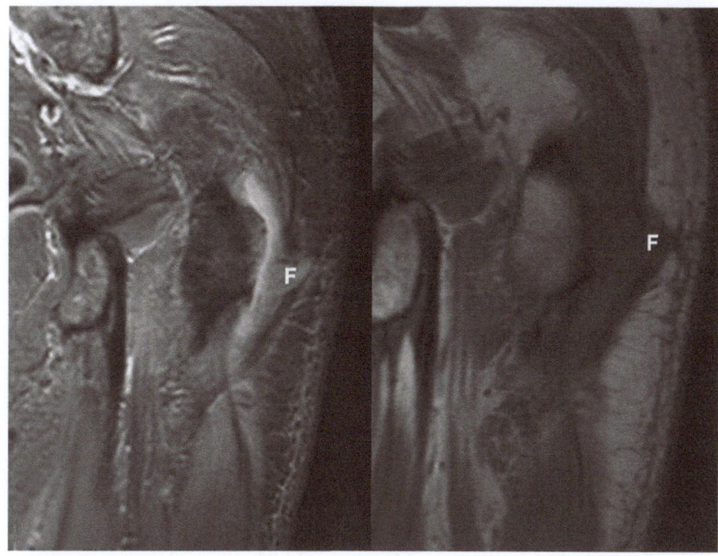

Fig. 19.2. AP pelvis and proximal femur MRI scan of a 71-year old man with a infected left total hip replacement. Joint-aspiration cultures are negative. The patient developed a skin fistula 15 days after the MRI. Note fluid periprosthetic extravasation and initial fistula (*F*) at MRI scan

trophils per high-power field are found in the periprosthetic tissue, but it is not possible to rule out infection when the number of neutrophils is less than five (Bori et al. 2007).

Total hip replacement deep infections can be sometimes difficult to diagnose but are always difficult to manage.

Total Hip Replacement Deep Infection Management

Deep infections are classified upon their first appearance respect to surgery, their presumed origin (local or hematogenous; Tsukayama et al. 1996) and the duration of symptoms and upon patient and limb health status (McPherson et al. 2002). Another empiric classification divides infected implants in infected loose implants and infected stable implants.

Acute infections (less than 4 weeks after surgery) and late but acute hematogenous infections (symptoms from less than 4 weeks) with stable implant can be managed with debridement alone and implant retention (changing only prosthetic head and cup inlay) with a reasonable percentage of success (Hanssen and Spangehl 2004; Crockarell et al. 1998). The same method must not be used in late chronic infections: only 15% success.

For deep late chronic periprosthetic infections there are four main treatment directions: one-stage revision, two-staged revision, resection arthroplasty and long-term suppression therapy. As a result of unsuccessful treatments an amputation can be necessary in more severe cases.

One-Stage Revision

One-stage revision or direct exchange arthroplasty consists of a single surgery to try to eradicate the deep infection with a reimplantation of a new prosthesis with antibiotic-loaded cement. One stage is very attractive. Every surgeon in the world instinctively would choose this method avoiding multiple surgeries and patients' suffering. One-stage revision has been popularized, in the eighties, by Buchholz with the introduction of antibiotic in acrylic bone cement (Buchholz et al. 1981). Buchholz described the results of 583 infected THR treated with a one-stage procedure, most of them without an accompanying oral antibiotic therapy. They had a success rate (no reinfection and no mechanical loosening) of 77% (Buchholz et al. 1984).

The same patients, eight years later, presented a 50% reinfection rate (Röttger 1986; Garvin and Hanssen 1995).

During the past two decades, one-stage revision techniques and indications have been refined achieving 83–84% success rates in wide series (Jackson and Schmalzried 2000; Raut et al. 1995). The use of antibiotic-loaded cement at high doses is mandatory (Hanssen and Rand 1999). The problem to load acrylic cement with antibiotic is that while less then 2 g of powdered antibiotics to 40 g bone cement do not reduce the compressive and tensile strength of the cement and more than 4.5 g of powdered antibiotics to 40 g bone cement do significantly affect its mechanical properties, the effects of doses between 2 g and 4.5 g, normally used in one-stage revision, are difficult to be assessed (Lautenschlager et al. 1976; Ger et al. 1977; Grauer et al. 1989). This could explain the high rate of loosening seen in different experiences with direct exchange arthroplasty (Buchholz et al. 1984; Röttger 1986; Garvin and Hanssen 1995). Another suspected explanation for the high rate of loosening could be a persistent low-grade infection.

Reading literature, one-stage procedure should be done if (Jackson and Schmalzried 2000; Langlais 2003)

- the pathogen has been isolated,
- it is not a polymicrobial infection or a bad pathogen infection (Pseudomonas aeruginosa, MRSA etc.),
- no unfavourable local conditions (wound complications, fibrosis, etc.),
- good general health of the patient,
- no excessive bone loss (need of bone-graft reconstruction).

And one stage should comprehend

- wide exposure, invasive and complete toilette of suspected tissues,
- antibiotic-loaded acrylic cemented prosthesis (dose?),
- hand-mixing, no vacuum,
- oral antibiotic therapy for a long period (at least 2 months).

Hanssen and Osmon (2000) try to find the percentage of patients with a good indication to direct exchange in a cohort of 37 patients with deep late infection using the nowadays criteria. After determination of culture data obtained preoperatively and additional exclusion by other selection criteria, there were only four (11%) patients with infected hip arthroplasties who would have been candidates for a direct exchange procedure. Moreover, in the overall group of 37 hips, 11 (30%) had an additional organism also identified by the cultures obtained from tissue samples removed during the prosthesis removal and one of the one-stage group had a methicillin-resistant coagulase-negative staphylococcus that, known before, would have excluded the patient from the direct exchange.

This means that if you want to do a one-stage procedure, first you must be very precise in isolating the pathogenic bacteria, then the patient must be in good health with a good not sclerotic bone and a good bone stock. Then you have to perform a radical debridement leaving enough bone to cement a new prosthesis and the patient must take a long-term antibiotic therapy. The overall success rate of all this: 80% if you do everything well and you consider also loosening.

Two-Stage Revision

Two-stage revision is the most used method of treatment for late deep THR infection and consists in two surgical steps. First step: implant removal, debridement and eventually placement of an antibiotic-loaded cement spacer. Second step: definitive reimplantation. There can be many differences in two stage revision procedures (Charlton et al. 2003; Takahira et al. 2003; Hsieh et al. 2004a,b, 2005; Yamamoto et al. 2003; Jahoda et al. 2003; Masri et al. 2007; Hofmann et al. 2005; Durbhakula et al. 2004; Etienne et al. 2003; Stockley et al. 2008; Diwanji et al. 2008): use/not use of a cement spacer, type of the spacer and kind/dose of antibiotic in spacer bone cement, interval between two steps, use of oral or parental antibiotics either in between, after reimplantation, cemented or cementless definitive revision etc.

As a matter of fact, if you do not use a spacer, you can have a good infection eradication rate but you will encounter surgical difficulties at reimplantation and bad clinical results as patient discomfort and shortening in 50% of the cases (Charlton et al. 2003; Hsieh et al. 2004).

The spacer can be self-made by the surgeon at the same time of surgery (Zawadsky et al. 2001) or can be pre-assembled out of the shelf spacer. Furthermore, the spacer can be an articulating spacer, a very high antibiotic-loaded cemented prosthesis with an intentionally loose cementing technique or, more frequently, an all cement partial prosthesis that can be made in different ways. We routinely use a self-made spacer reinforced by a Kirschner wire bended either at the top, as a buttress, to better hold a minimal weight-bearing. We try to make the spacer wider possible often resembling a proximal femoral epiphysis (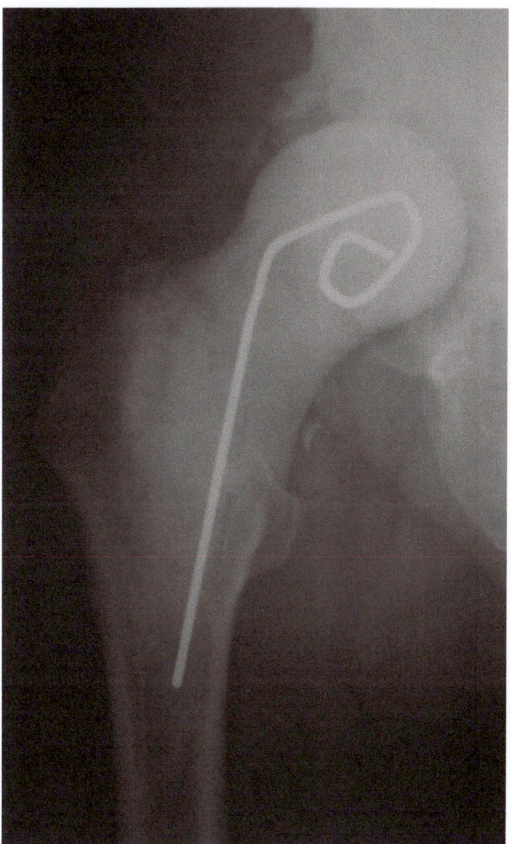 Fig. 19.3). More recently we bend the wire also at the bottom to facilitate spacer »en-bloc« removal.

Fig. 19.3. AP X-ray of a right hip of a patient after spacer insertion. Note the anatomical shape of the spacer and the bended Kirschner wire

Types and doses of antibiotic used in bone cement are very different in literature (Charlton et al. 2003; Takahira et al. 2003; Hsieh et al. 2004a,b, 2005; Yamamoto et al. 2003; Jahoda et al. 2003; Masri et al. 2007; Hofmann et al. 2005; Durbhakula et al. 2004; Etienne et al. 2003; Stockley et al. 2008; Diwanji et al. 2008). Antibiotic dose can be as low as 0.5 g of gentamicin in 40 g of bone cement (Leunig et al. 1998) and as high as 8 g of different antibiotics in 40 g of bone cement (Hsieh et al. 2004). High doses are recommended to get a maximum antibiotic local concentration. The problem of cement mechanical strength is much less important than in one-stage procedure. Most used antibiotics are gentamicin, vancomycin and tobramicyn. The combined use of tobramicyn and vancomycin results in a better antibiotics diffusion (Penner et al. 1996). When possible and upon cultures different antibiotics are used (Hsieh et al. 2004b).

Time between the two surgical procedures is essential. A brief period of time demonstrated very bad results (Colyerm and Capello 1994). Recommended period is more than 8 weeks and depends on inflammation marker negativization and antibiotic therapy. We use to leave at least one month, without antibiotic, between CRP negativization and reimplantation.

Another very important factor in two-stage procedure, as it is in one stage, is a prolonged antibiotic therapy for at least 6 weeks, and started intravenously, after first step. We use at least a one-month antibiotic therapy also after reimplantation. The none-use of antibiotic therapy reduces the change of success (Stockley et al. 2008).

The definitive replacement in two-steps procedure can be cemented or cementless as the surgeon choice. It does not seem so crucial nowadays to choose a cemented prosthesis as definitive implant in two-stage procedures.

If all recommendations are followed, the expected infection eradication is 94–98% (Charlton et al. 2003; Takahira et al. 2003; Hsieh et al. 2004a,b, 2005; Yamamoto et al. 2003; Jahoda et al. 2003; Masri et al. 2007; Hofmann et al. 2005; Durbhakula et al. 2004; Etienne et al. 2003; Stockley et al. 2008; Diwanji et al. 2008).

Furthermore, the two-stage procedure is the only one applicable if bone graft for reconstruction

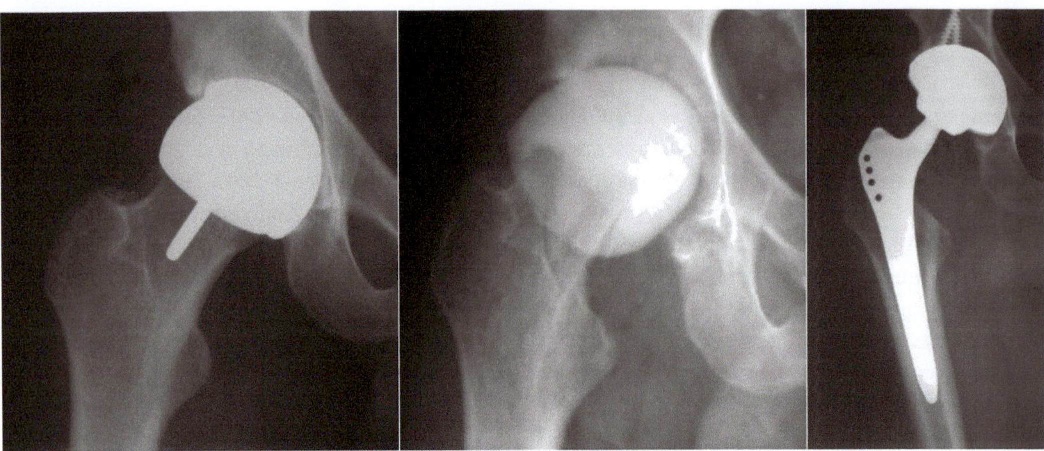

Fig. 19.4. X-ray views on a right hip in a patient with a resurfacing infection. Before, during and after a two-stage procedure. Note the femoral cup spacer without femoral canal violation

is needed. In this case, vancomycin can be added to donor bone graft (Buttaro et al. 2005).

In case of resurfacing infection it also seem reasonable to do a two-stage procedure with a shaped cup spacer instead of a one-stage procedure violating the un-opened femoral canal (Fig. 19.4).

Conclusion

One-stage procedure or direct exchange in infected total hip replacement has very limited indications. The wide and uncontrolled use of this procedure reduces infection eradication percentage. Early loosening is another complication that can be encountered.

Two-stage procedure is a more demanding procedure but has wider indications and, if good conducted, a higher percentage of success.

References

Barrack RL, Harris WH (1993) The value of aspiration of the hip joint before revision total hip arthroplasty. J Bone Joint Surg Am 75-A: 66–76

Bongartz T, Halligan CS, Osmon DR, Reinalda MS, Bamlet WR, Crowson CS, Hanssen AD, Matteson EL (2008 Dec 15) Incidence and risk factors of prosthetic joint infection after total hip or knee replacement in patients with rheumatoid arthritis. Arthritis Rheum. 59(12):1713-1720.

Bori G, Soriano A, García S, Mallofré C, Riba J, Mensa J (2007) Usefulness of histological analysis for predicting the presence of microorganisms at the time of reimplantation after hip resection arthroplasty for the treatment of infection. J Bone Joint Surg Am 89: 1232–1237

Bottner F, Sculco TP (2001) Infection in revision total hip arthroplasty. Tech Orthop 16: 310–322

Bottner F, Wegner A, Winkelmann W, Becker K, Erren M, Götze C (2007) Interleukin-6, procalcitonin and TNF-α. Markers of peri-prosthetic infection following total joint replacement. J Bone Joint Surg 89-B: 94–99

Buchholz HW, Elson RA, Engelbrecht E et al. (1981) Management of deep infection of total hip replacement. J Bone Joint Surg 63B: 342–353

Buchholz HW, Elson RA, Heinert K (1984) Antibiotic-loaded acrylic cement: Current Concept. CORR 190: 96–108

Buttaro MA, Pusso R, Piccaluga F (2005) Vancomycin-supplemented impacted bone allografts in infected hip arthroplasty. Two-stage revision results. J Bone Joint Surg Br 87-B: 314–319

Charlton WP, Hozack WJ, Teloken MA, Rao R, Bissett GA (2003) Complications associated with reimplantation after Girdlestone arthroplasty. Clin Orthop Rel Res 407: 119–126

Charnley J (1972) Postoperative infection after total hip replacement with special reference to air contamination in the operating room. Clin Orthop Relat Res 87: 167–187

Colyerm R, Capello WN (1994) Surgical treatment of the infected hip implant. two-stage reimplantation with a one-month interval. CORR 298: 15–19

Crockarell JR Jr, Hanssen AD, Osmon DR et al. (1998) Treatment of infection with debridement and retention of the components following hip arthroplasty. J Bone Joint Surg 80A: 1306–1313

Di Cesare PE, Chang E, Preston CF, Liu C-J (2005) Serum interleukin-6 as a marker of periprosthetic infection following total hip and knee arthroplasty. J Bone Joint Surg 87-A: 1921–1927

Diwanji SR, Kong IK, Park YH, Cho SG, Song EK, Yoon TR (2008) Two-stage reconstruction of infected hip joints. J Arthroplasty 23: 656–661

Durbhakula SM, Czajka J, Fuchs MD, Uhl RL (2004) Spacer endoprosthesis for the treatment of infected total hip arthroplasty. J Arthroplasty 19: 760–767

Etienne G, Waldman B, Rajadhyaksha AD, Ragland PS, Mont MA (2003) Use of a functional temporary prosthesis in a two-stage approach to infection at the site of a total hip arthroplasty. J Bone Joint Surg Am 85 (Suppl 4): 94–96

Fitzgerald RH, Bechtol CO, Eftekhar N, Nelson JP (1979) Reduction of deep sepsis after total hip replacement. Arch Surg 7: 803–804

Garvin KL, Hanssen AD (1995) Infection after total hip arthroplasty: past, present and future. J Bone Joint Surg Am 77: 1576–1588

Ger E, Dall D, Miles T, Forder A (1977) Bone cement and antibiotics. S Afr Med J 51: 276–279

Grauer JD, Amstutz HC, O'Carroll PF et al. (1989) Resection arthroplasty of the hip. J Bone Joint Surg Am 71: 669–678

Gristina AG, Costerton JW (1984) Bacteria-laden biofilms: A hazard to orthopedic prostheses. Infections Surg 3: 655–662

Gristina AG, Naylor PT, Meador TL (1991) Biomaterial surface domains: Bacterial versus tissue cells. In: Bender M (ed) Interfacial phenomena in biological systems. Marcel Dekker, New York, pp 105–136

Hansenn AD, Spangehl MJ (2004) Treatment of the infected hip replacement. Clin Orthop 420: 63–71

Hanssen AD, Osmon DR (2000) Assessment of patient selection criteria for treatment of the infected hip arthroplasty. CORR 381: 91–100

Hanssen AD, Rand JA (1999) Evaluation and treatment of infection at the site of a total hip or knee arthroplasty. Instr Course Lect 48: 111–122

Hofmann AA, Goldberg TD, Tanner AM, Cook TM (2005) Ten-year experience using an articulating antibiotic cement hip spacer for the treatment of chronically infected total hip. J Arthroplasty 20: 874–879

Hsieh PH, Chen LH, Chen CH, Lee MS, Yang WE, Shih CH (2004b) Two-stage revision hip arthroplasty for infection with a custom-made, antibiotic-loaded cement prosthesis as an interim spacer. J Trauma 56: 1247–1252

Hsieh PH, Shih CH, Chang YH, Lee MS, Shih HN, Yang WE (2004a) Two-stage revision hip arthroplasty for infection: comparison between the interim use of antibiotic-loaded cement beads and a spacer prosthesis. J Bone Joint Surg Am 86-A: 1989–1997

Hsieh PH, Shih CH, Chang YH, Lee MS, Yang WE, Shih HN (2005) Two-stage revision with an antibiotic-loaded interim cement prosthesis followed by reconstruction with allograft. J Bone Joint Surg Br 87-B: 770–775

Jackson WO, Schmalzried TP (2000) Limited role of direct exchange arthroplasty in the treatment of infected total hip replacements. Clin Orthop 381: 101–105

Jahoda D, Sosna A, Landor I, Vavrik P, Pokorny D (2003) Cannulated spacer in the treatment of deep infection of total hip artroplasty using a two-stage reimplantation. Operat Orthop Traumatol 15: 57–69

Johnston C, Kerr J, O'Byrne J, Eustace S (2007) MRI as a problem-solving tool in unexplained failed total hip replacement following conventional assessment. Skeletal Radiol 36: 955–961

Langlais F (2003) can we improve the results of revision arthroplasty for infected total hip replacement? J Bone Joint Surg 85-B: 637–640

Lautenschlager EP, Marshall GW, Marks KE, Schwartz J, Nelson CL (1976) Mechanical strength of acrylic bone cements impregnated with antibiotics. J Biomed Mater Res 10: 837–45

M. Leunig, E. Chosa, M. Speck, R. Ganz (1998) A cement spacer for two-stage revision of infected implants of the hip joint. International Orthopaedics (SICOT) 22: 209–214

Marculescu CE, Berbari EF, Hanssen AD, Steckelberg JM, Osmon DR (2005) Prosthetic joint infection diagnosed postoperatively by intraoperative culture. CORR 439: 38–42

Masri BA, Panagiotopoulos KP, Greidanus NV, Garbuz DS, Duncan CP (2007) Cementless two-stage exchange arthroplasty for infection after total hip arthroplasty. J Arthroplasty 22: 72–78

McDowell A, Patrick S (2005) Evaluation of nonculture methods for the detection of prosthetic hip biofilms. CORR 437: 74–82

McPherson EJ, Woodson C, Holtom P, Roidis N, Shufelt C, Patzakis M (2002) Periprosthetic total hip infection. Outcomes using a staging system. CORR 403: 8–15

Nguyen LL, Nelson CL, Saccente M, Smeltzer MS, Wassell DL, McLaren SG (2002) Detecting bacterial colonization of implanted orthopaedic devices by ultrasonication. CORR 403: 29–37

Penner MJ, Masri BA, Duncan CP (1996) Elution characteristics of vancomycin and tobramycin combined in acrylic bone-cement. J Arthroplasty 11: 939–944

Raut VV, Siney PD, Wroblewski BM (1995) One-stage revision of total hip arthroplasty for deep infection. Clin Orthop 321: 202–207

Reinartz P, Mumme T, Hermanns B et al. (2005) Radionuclide imaging of the painful hip arthroplasty positron-emission tomography versus triple-phase bone scanning. J Bone Joint Surg 87-B: 465–470

Ridgeway S, Wilson J, Charlet A et al. (2005) Infection of the surgical site after arthroplasty of the hip. J Bone Joint Surg Br 87-B: 844–850

Ritter MA, Olberding EM, Malinzak RA (2007) Ultraviolet lighting during orthopaedic surgery and the rate of infection. J Bone Joint Surg Am 89: 1935–1940

Röttger J (1986) Symposium: antibiotic-impregnated acrylic composites. Contemp Orthop 12: 85–135

Spangehl MJ, Masri BA, O'Connell JX et al. (1999) Prospective analysis of preoperative and intraoperative investigations for the diagnosis of infection at the side of two hundred and two revision total hip arthroplasties. J Bone Joint Surg Am 81: 672–683

Stockley I, Mockford BJ, Hoad-Reddick A, Norman P (2008) The use of two-stage exchange arthroplasty with depot antibiotics in the absence of longterm antibiotic therapy in infected total hip replacement. J Bone Joint Surg Br 90-B: 145–148

Stockley I, Mockford BJ, Hoad-Reddick A, Norman P (2008) The use of two-stage exchange arthroplasty with depot antibiotics in the absence of longterm antibiotic therapy in infected total hip replacement. J Bone J Surg Am 90-A: 145–148

Takahira N, Itoman M, Higashi K, Uchiyama K, Miyabe M, Naruse K (2003) Treatment outcome of two-stage revision total hip arthroplasty for infected hip arthroplasty using antibiotic-impregnated cement spacer. J Orthop Sci 8: 26–31

Tsukayama DT, Estrada R, Gustilo RB (1996) Infection after total hip arthroplasty. A study of the treatment of one hundred and six infections. J Bone Joint Surg Am 78: 512–523

Wilson J, Charlett A, Leong G, McDougall C, Duckworth G (2008) Rates of surgical site infection after hip replacement as a hospital performance indicator: analysis of data from the English Mandatory Surveillance System. Infect Control Hosp Epidemiol 29: 219–226

Yamamoto K, Miyagawa N, Masaoka T, Katori Y, Shishido T, Imakiire A (2003) Clinical effectiveness of antibiotic-impregnated cement spacewrs for the treatment of infected implants of the hip joint. J Orthop Sci 8: 823–828

Zawadsky MW, Pearle AD, Sculco TP (2001) Three techniques for the fabrication of cement spacers in the treatment of an infected total hip arthroplasty. Tech Orthop 16: 330–335

Subject Index

Printing: Ten Brink, Meppel, The Netherlands
Binding: Stürtz, Würzburg, Germany